*The Natural Medicine Guide to*

# DEPRESSION

**Books by Stephanie Marohn**

*Natural Medicine First Aid Remedies*

*The Natural Medicine Guide to Autism*

*The Natural Medicine Guide to Bipolar Disorder*

THE HEALTHY MIND GUIDES

# The Natural Medicine Guide to

# DEPRESSION

## Stephanie Marohn

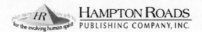

HAMPTON ROADS
PUBLISHING COMPANY, INC.
for the evolving human spirit

Cover design by Bookwrights Design
Cover art © 2002 Loyd Chapplow
Interior MediClip image © 2003 Williams and Wilkins.
All rights reserved.
Acupuncture meridian illustrations by Anne L. Louque

Hampton Roads Publishing Company, Inc.
1125 Stoney Ridge Road
Charlottesville, VA 22902

434-296-2772
fax: 434-296-5096
e-mail: hrpc@hrpub.com
www.hrpub.com

If you are unable to order this book from your local
bookseller, you may order directly from the publisher.
Call 1-800-766-8009, toll-free.
ISBN 1-57174-292-1

Library of Congress Cataloging-in-Publication Data

Marohn, Stephanie.
  The natural medicine guide to depression / by Stephanie Marohn.
    p. ; cm. -- (The healthy mind guides)
Includes bibliographical references and index.
  ISBN 1-57174-292-1 (alk. paper)
  1. Depression, Mental--Alternative treatment.
  [DNLM: 1. Complementary Therapies--Popular Works. 2.
Depressive Disorder--therapy--Popular Works. WM 171 M354n 2002]
I. Title. II. Series.
  RC537 .M373 2002
  616.85'2706--dc21

                                          2002153238

10 9 8 7 6 5 4 3 2 1
Printed on acid-free paper in Canada

# THE HEALTHY 🙢 MIND GUIDES

**THE HEALTHY MIND GUIDES** are a series of books offering original research and treatment options for reversing or ameliorating several so-called mental disorders, written by noted health journalist and author Stephanie Marohn. The series' focus is the natural medicine approach, a refreshing and hopeful outlook based on treating individual needs rather than medical labels, and addressing the underlying imbalances—biological, psychological, emotional, and spiritual.

Each book in the series offers the very latest information about the possible causes of each disorder, and presents a wide range of effective, practical therapies drawn from extensive interviews with physicians and other practitioners who are innovators in their respective fields. Case studies throughout the books illustrate the applications of these therapies, and numerous resources are provided for readers who want to seek treatment.

♣

*To those who are struggling in the darkness of depression*

# Acknowledgments

My deep gratitude to the doctors and other healing professionals who provided information on their work for the natural medicine treatment chapters in the book. I am very appreciative of all the time and energy you so generously gave. Specifically, my thanks to:

Johannes Beckmann, M.D.
Ira J. Golchehreh, L.Ac., O.M.D.
Patricia Kaminski
Dietrich Klinghardt, M.D., Ph.D.
Reverend Leon S. LeGant
Thomas M. Rau, M.D.
Judyth Reichenberg-Ullman, N.D., L.C.S.W.
Tony Roffers, Ph.D.
Malidoma Patrice Somé, Ph.D.
Zannah Steiner, C.M.P., R.M.T.
Bradford S. Weeks, M.D.

Great thanks to my brilliant physicians Dr. Ira Golchehreh and Dr. Thomas Rau for taking such good care of me.

Loving gratitude to my dear, dear friends Donna Canali, Mella Mincberg, and Moli Steinert for all that we share and for the sheer pleasure of your company.

Thank-you to my parents for your lifelong belief in my abilities and all the support you've given me over the years.

Continued gratitude to Nancy Gallenson for celebration, support, and inspired ballet classes.

My appreciation to Sue Trowbridge and Dorothy Anderson for all your hard work transcribing many interviews, and to Adrienne Fodor of the Institute for Health and Healing Resource Center in San Francisco for research assistance.

And finally, thanks yet again to my friend and editor Richard Leviton.

# Contents

# Introduction

We in the United States and other countries in the developed world are in the midst of a mental health crisis. The psychiatric treatment methods we have been using are not working, as is clear from the dire statistics on mental illness. Here are just a few:

- Mental illness is the second leading cause of disability and premature mortality in the U.S. and other developed countries.[1]

- 4 of the 10 leading causes of disability in the U.S. and other developed countries are mental disorders—major depression, bipolar disorder, obsessive-compulsive disorder, or schizophrenia.[2]

- 5.4 percent of adults in the U.S. have a serious mental illness (defined as "substantial interference with one or more major life activities"; less severe mental illness is not included in this statistic).[3]

- 1 in 4 hospital admissions in the U.S. in 1998 were psychiatric admissions.[4]

- $148 billion = the total cost of mental health services in the U.S. in 1990[5] ($69 billion in direct costs for mental health treatment and rehabilitation, and $79 billion in the indirect costs of lost productivity at work, school, or home due to disability or death).

A large reason why treatment of mental illness has a poor success record and is costing more all the time is because the overwhelming emphasis is placed on pharmaceutical drugs. Not everyone in the psychiatric field is happy with the ever-increasing governance of psychopharmacology (the science of drugs used to affect behavior and emotional states). Here is what one psychiatrist had to say about it. In December 1998, in a letter of resignation to the president of the American Psychiatric Association (APA), Loren R. Mosher, M.D., former official of the National Institute of Mental Health (NIMH), wrote:[6]

> After nearly three decades as a member, it is with a mixture of pleasure and disappointment that I submit this letter of resignation from the American Psychiatric Association. The major reason for this action is my belief that I am actually resigning from the American Psychopharmacological Association. . . .
>
> At this point in history, in my view, psychiatry has been almost completely bought out by the drug companies. . . .
>
> We condone and promote the widespread overuse and misuse of toxic chemicals that we know have serious long term effects. . . .

While psychiatric drugs (prescription drugs used for mental illnesses) may control certain disorders, and in some instances save lives, they do not cure the disorder, and they often compound the person's problems with disturbing side effects in the short term and the risk of permanent damage in the long term. If we are going to solve the current mental health crisis, we are going to have to turn to other approaches to treatment.

The state of affairs in psychiatric treatment is reflected in the focus of quite a few of the books on mental illness aimed at the general public. The help they offer involves information for the patient on coping with hospitalization; for family members on how to live with the illness in a loved one; and on how to work with side effects of antidepressants and other psychopharmaceuticals (psychiatric drugs)—that is, what other drugs you can take to reduce those effects.

The focus of *The Natural Medicine Guide to Depression* is healing from depression, not learning to live with it. The book explores the causes of depression and offers a range of treatment approaches to address those causes and truly restore health. Only by treating the underlying causes of depression, rather than suppressing the symptoms as most drugs do, can lasting recovery be achieved. And only by considering the well-being of the mind and spirit in addition to the body can comprehensive healing take place.

All of the therapies covered here approach the treatment of depression in this way. They all also share the characteristic of tailoring treatment to the individual, which is another essential element for a successful outcome. No two people, even with the same diagnosis, have exactly the same imbalances causing their problems.

With the increase in the number of people who are using natural therapies, the public has become more aware of this medical approach. When many people think of natural medicine, however, they think of supplements or herbal remedies available over the counter. While these products can be highly beneficial, natural medicine is far more than that. Natural therapies are those that operate according to holistic principles, meaning treating the whole person rather than an isolated part or symptom and using natural treatments that "Do no harm" and support or restore the body's natural ability to heal itself. Natural medicine involves a way of looking at healing that is dramatically different from the conventional medical model. It does not mimic that model by

**This book explores the causes of depression and offers a range of treatment approaches to address those causes and truly restore health. Only by treating the underlying causes of depression, rather than suppressing the symptoms as most drugs do, can lasting recovery be achieved.**

merely substituting an herb for an antidepressant. Instead, it uses the comprehensive approach just described, which offers you the very real possibility of curing your depression.

I speak from personal experience. I struggled with depression my whole life. It was always there to some degree, sometimes worse than at others. Like two-thirds of the people who suffer from depression, I never sought treatment for it, although I began psychotherapy in my twenties to try to sort out my life and continued it off and on for the next ten years. While psychotherapy was tremendously valuable to me, it didn't solve my depression problem.

Many natural medicine doctors have told me that depressed patients usually come to them for other reasons and discover that treatment gets rid of their depression too. I was no exception. And many people also discover that their depression has no one cause. I too learned that. The therapies that provided the solution for me were traditional Chinese medicine (both acupuncture and Chinese herbs), constitutional homeopathy, and having my mercury fillings replaced. I used them in that order, but it was not conscious; it just happened that way. It was as if I was peeling the layers of an onion, with each layer being another imbalance I needed to uncover and correct.

Transpersonal psychotherapy led me to the last missing piece in my full recovery: the spiritual. Or to stay with the metaphor, you could say that I reached the center of the onion. I had already taken care of the body and mind in many ways, but my depression didn't completely disappear until I found my way back to a connection with spirit. Finally, I feel that my body, mind, and spirit are in harmony.

I tell you my story to give you an idea of how the therapies in this book can be used together, to peel the layers of your depression.

Before I tell you a little about what's in the book, I would just like to say a few words about the terms *mental illness* and *mental disorders,* or *brain disorders* as they are more currently labeled. All of these terms reflect the disconnection between body and mind—spirit is not even in the picture—in conventional medical treatment. The newer term, brain disorders, reflects the biochemical model of causality that currently dominates the medical profession.

I use the terms *mental illness* and *mental disorders* in this book because there is no easy substitute that reflects the true body-mind-spirit nature of these conditions. While I may use these terms, I in no way mean to suggest that the causes of the disorders lie solely in the mind. The same is true for the title of the series of which this book is a part: The Healthy Mind Guides. The name serves to distinguish the subject area, but it is healthy mind, body, and spirit—wholeness—that is the focus of these books.

While I'm at it, I may as well dispense with one last linguistic issue. As natural medicine effects profound healing, rather than simply controlling symptoms, I prefer the term *natural medicine* over *alternative medicine*. This medical model is not "other"—it is a primary form of medicine. The term *holistic medicine* reflects this as well, in that it signals the natural medicine approach of treating the whole person, rather than the parts.

As I said, the focus of this book is on comprehensive treatments. There are a number of books on the market that cover natural self-help medicines that aid in alleviating depression, such as the herbal remedy St. John's wort. While various of these remedies have shown benefit in alleviating depression, they do not address the underlying causes and, for that reason, I don't cover them in this book, which is dedicated to the deeper treatments. (For self-help treatments for depression, see my book *Natural Medicine First Aid Remedies,* Hampton Roads, 2001.)

Part 1 of *The Natural Medicine Guide to Depression* covers the basics of depression: what it is, who gets it, and what causes it. The natural medicine view of depression is that it is a multicausal disorder, with a variety of contributing factors.

Part 2 of the book covers a range of natural medicine treatments for depression. The material presented here is based on research and interviews with physicians and other healing professionals who are leaders and pioneers in their respective fields. This is original information, not derivative material gleaned from secondary sources. The therapeutic techniques of these highly skilled and experienced healers are explained in detail and illustrated with case studies (the names of patients throughout the book have been changed). Contact information for the practitioners whose work is presented appears in appendix B: Resources.

May the information in this book help you find your way out of depression.

# Natural Medicine Therapies Covered in Part 2

| CHAPTER | HEALTH PRACTITIONER | THERAPIES |
|---|---|---|
| 3 | Dietrich Klinghardt, M.D., Ph.D. | APN (Applied Psycho-Neurobiology) |
| | | ART (Autonomic Response Testing) |
| | | Chelation/heavy metal detoxification |
| | | Family Systems Therapy |
| | | NAET (allergy elimination) |
| | | Neural Therapy |
| | | Thought Field Therapy |
| 4 | Thomas M. Rau, M.D. | Biological medicine |
| | Bradford S. Weeks, M.D. | Anthroposophic medicine |
| 5 | Ira J. Golchehreh, L.Ac., O.M.D. | Traditional Chinese medicine |
| | | Acupuncture |
| | | Herbal medicine |
| 6 | Judyth Reichenberg-Ullman, N.D., L.C.S.W. | Constitutional homeopathy |
| 7 | Patricia Kaminski | Flower essence therapy |
| 8 | Zannah Steiner, C.M.P., R.M.T. | CranioSacral therapy |
| | | Visceral Manipulation |
| | | SomatoEmotional Release |
| | | Process-Oriented Counseling |
| 9 | Tony Roffers, Ph.D. | Seemorg Matrix Work |
| | Johannes Beckmann, M.D. | Psychosomatic medicine |
| 10 | Malidoma Patrice Somé, Ph.D. | Shamanic healing |
| | Rev. Leon S. LeGant | Spiritual/psychic healing |

# PART I

# *The Basics of Depression*

# 1 What Is Depression and Who Suffers from It?

Depression falls into the category of mood disorders, also known as affective disorders. It encompasses a continuum of disturbance in thoughts, feelings, behaviors, and physical health, with the prevailing characteristic of persistent sadness and despair. While some people experience depression to the point that they can no longer function in their lives, others may not even realize that they are depressed. An estimated twelve million people in the United States are not aware that they are suffering from depression,[7] and 80 percent of primary care patients actually fit the criteria for a diagnosis of major depression.[8]

Melancholia, a former term for depression, has plagued humankind for at least as long as recorded history, and likely from the beginning of human existence. Written accounts of depression date back to 2500 B.C., with an ancient Egyptian papyrus relating a man's despair and sense of emptiness as he contemplates suicide.[9] One way of explaining the presence of mood in the human spirit is to regard it as an evolutionary adaptation.[10] A depression in mood, for example, pulls us back from engagement with life, which we may need at that moment to keep us safe or to give us time to gain a perspective.

Viewed in this light, one might say that there is a tremendous need today for safety and perspective, given that depression is a worldwide epidemic. This point gains validity when one considers

## In Their Own Words

*"What's really diabolical about it is that if there were a pill over there, ten feet from me, that you could guarantee would lift me out of it, it would be too much trouble to go get it."*

—Dick Cavett,
on his severe depression[14]

the complexity, toxicity, and stress of modern life and the physical, psychological/emotional, and spiritual causes of depression, as discussed in chapter 2 and throughout the book.

In the United States alone, thirty million people are taking Prozac, which is now in the top ten most prescribed drugs.[11]

That translates to nearly one in ten people. One in eight adolescents and one in thirty-three children overall suffer from depression. One in four women will have clinical depression in their lifetime—twice the rate for men. (These rates reflect reported cases. The rate for men may actually be equal to that of women as societal factors contribute to men not seeking help.) Depression cuts across all ages, with more than one in six people over the age of 65 afflicted.[12]

While the devastation of depression cannot be measured solely in dollar amounts, its economic cost illuminates its far-reaching reverberations. The annual cost of depressive disorders in the United States is $43 billion, a total of the costs of direct treatment, absenteeism, lost productivity, and mortality.[13]

Another tragic set of statistics reflects the profound human loss resulting from depression. A study by the World Health Organization (WHO) and the Harvard School of Public Health reveals that by the year 2020 depression will be the single leading cause of death around the globe.[15]

The risk of suicide is 30 times greater among people with depression than in the general population.[16] In the United States alone, there are 30,000 suicides every year.[17] Suicide among the teen population has increased 300 percent in the past 30 years.[18] Among children between the ages of 10 and 14, the rate of suicide has more than doubled in the last 10 years. For youth between the ages of 15 and 24, suicide is now the third leading cause of death. For college students, it is the second leading cause.[19]

While the statistics on depression and its effects are grim, they reflect the fact that only one in three people with a major mood disorder seek help,[20] and 50 percent of people with clinical depression turn to their primary care physician, who may or may not have the training needed to provide true assistance.[21] The dismal nature of the statistics also reflects the fact that the vast majority of those who seek help for their depression

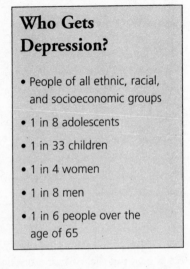

## Who Gets Depression?

- People of all ethnic, racial, and socioeconomic groups
- 1 in 8 adolescents
- 1 in 33 children
- 1 in 4 women
- 1 in 8 men
- 1 in 6 people over the age of 65

are receiving conventional treatment, which does not have a good success rate (as the epidemic proportions of depression verify).

The overwhelming emphasis in the conventional approach to depression is on antidepressant drugs. Despite the fact that psychotherapy is cited as a primary component in WHO and APA (American Psychiatric Association) standards for depression treatment, its use accounts for just eight percent of the money expended in treating depression.[22]

Unfortunately, the effectiveness of antidepressants is greatly overrated. In disregard of disturbing side effects and of research showing that they do not work for a third of the people who take them, and do no better than placebos for another third,[23] these drugs continue to be dispensed widely and to be regarded as the panacea for depression.

While in some cases of chronic severe depression, they may provide an important intervention to save a life, antidepressants are handed out far too freely. The prescription flurry is now extending to increasing numbers of children, despite the fact that Prozac and similar antidepressants are approved by the Food and Drug Administration (FDA) only for use in patients over the age of 18.[24] Even for those people who get welcome relief from antidepressants, it is important to keep in mind that they are not getting a cure for their depression, in that the drugs do not address the underlying factors that caused the depression in the first place.

Fortunately, there is a way out of this current state of affairs. The statistics of depression will change to a far more positive picture as more people learn about and gain access to natural medicine approaches to the disorder, which make profound and lasting recovery from depression a strong possibility. Meanwhile, the present statistics should put the medical profession on alert that changes need to happen in regard to the treatment of depression. The statistics also serve another important function: to highlight how important it is to determine if you are suffering from depression and to get help.

## Types of Depression

The common subcategories of depression are major depressive disorder, dysthymia, and seasonal affective disorder. Major depressive disorder is also known as clinical depression, major depression, major affective disorder, and unipolar disorder. Dysthymia, being chronic moderate depression, is the type that many people fail to recognize as a mood disorder. Seasonal affective disorder, or SAD, results from the reduced light of the winter season, which explains why it is known colloquially as "the winter blues."

 Bipolar disorder (formerly known as manic-depression) is another mood disorder involving depression. It is not covered in this book because

---

*This translation by Bika Reed can be found in her book, *Rebel in the Soul* (Rochester, VT: Inner Traditions International, 1987)

another book in *The Healthy Mind Guide* series is devoted to that subject. See the author's *The Natural Medicine Guide to Bipolar Disorder* (Hampton Roads, 2003).

A holistic approach does not use such diagnoses to determine the appropriate treatment course, focusing instead on the particular manifestations and underlying imbalances in the individual patient. Many people receive these labels, however, so it's helpful to know to what they refer.

For a diagnosis of major depressive disorder, according to the *Diagnostic and Statistical Manual of Mental Disorders*, Fourth Edition (*DSM-IV*), the APA's diagnostic bible for psychiatric disorders, a person must have one or more major depressive episodes, which are defined as depressed mood or loss of interest lasting at least two weeks and accompanied by at least four other symptoms of depression (see lists that follow). For dysthymia, the person must have experienced a depressed mood for more days than not over at least a two-year period, accompanied by other symptoms of depression, but the whole does not fit the diagnostic picture of major depressive disorder. SAD is depression that occurs on a seasonal basis and does not fit the criteria for any of the other depressive disorders that involve a seasonal pattern.[25]

> *The statistics of depression will change to a far more positive picture as more people learn about and gain access to natural medicine approaches to the disorder, which make profound and lasting recovery from depression a strong possibility.*

The following are symptoms of depression:[26]

- persistent sadness
- significantly reduced interest or pleasure
- significant change in weight or appetite

# Famous People with Mood Disorders

The following are among the well-known people who were diagnosed with or believed to have had a mood disorder:[27]

Alexander the Great
Napolean Bonaparte
Winston Churchill
Diana, Princess of Wales
Sigmund Freud
Abraham Lincoln
Sir Isaac Newton
Theodore Roosevelt

George Frederick Handel
Janet Jackson
Elton John
Gustav Mahler
Charlie Parker
Cole Porter
Bonnie Raitt
Robert Schumann

**Actors**

Marlon Brando
Richard Dreyfuss
Patty Duke
Audrey Hepburn
Ashley Judd
Margo Kidder
Roseanne
Winona Ryder
Damon Wayans

**Artists**

Michelangelo
Georgia O'Keeffe
Jackson Pollock
Vincent van Gogh

**Composers/Musicians/Singers**

Hector Berlioz
Ray Charles
Frederic Chopin
Kurt Cobain
Natalie Cole

**Writers**

Hans Christian Andersen
Honoré de Balzac
Michael Crichton
Charles Dickens
Emily Dickinson
William Faulkner
F. Scott Fitzgerald
Ernest Hemingway
Anne Sexton
Neil Simon
William Styron
Leo Tolstoy
Walt Whitman
Tennessee Williams
Virginia Woolf

**Athletes**

Oksana Baiul
Greg Louganis
Monica Seles
Darryl Strawberry

- insomnia or oversleeping
- restlessness, agitation, or lethargy
- fatigue or lack of energy
- feelings of worthlessness or excessive or inappropriate guilt
- problems thinking, concentrating, or making decisions
- recurrent thoughts of death or suicide

## In Their Own Words

*"Until one has experienced a debilitating severe depression it is hard to understand the feelings of those who have it....It was the worse experience of my life. More terrible even than watching my wife die of cancer. I am ashamed to admit that my depression felt worse than her death but it is true."*
—Lewis Wolpert, author of *Malignant Sadness*[28]

While these are the symptoms for diagnosis according to *DSM-IV* criteria, anxiety, even extreme anxiety, is another common symptom of depression.[29]

Since this fact is not well known, the anxiety can serve to mask the depressive disorder. Other symptoms of depression include:

- pessimism
- feelings of emptiness
- feelings of helplessness
- irritability or anger without apparent cause
- tearfulness or excessive crying
- withdrawal from social activities
- loss of interest in formerly pleasurable activities, including sex
- desire for solitude
- unexplained aches and pains

Depression can be a corollary of other medical conditions (see chapter 2) and there is a comorbidity factor with substance

## In Their Own Words

*"Most days, when I was depressed, I just felt a serious lack of energy and connectedness. On medium-bad days I walked around in a quiet state of desperation. When the depression was really bad, well, it was really bad."*

—Catherine Carrigan, author of Healing Depression[32]

abuse, eating disorders, and obsessive-compulsive disorder (OCD). Comorbidity means that two disorders exist together. In the case of substance abuse in relation to depression, for example, alcoholism is a factor in 30 percent of all suicides.[30]

In addition to identifying whether or not you or a loved one is suffering from depression, it is also important to be aware of the warning signs of suicide, so you are forewarned and can act to prevent this tragedy from happening if the signs begin to manifest. A family history of suicide or a previous suicide attempt places one at increased risk of suicide. In addition, the warning signs of suicide are:[31]

• feelings of hopelessness, worthlessness, anguish, or desperation

• withdrawal from people and activities

• preoccupation with death or morbid subjects

• sudden mood improvement or increased activity after a period of depression

• increase in risk-taking behaviors

• buying a gun

• putting affairs in order

• thinking, talking, or writing about a plan for committing suicide

If you think that you or someone you know is in danger of attempting suicide, call your doctor or a suicide hotline or get help from another qualified source. Know that there is help and, though it may be difficult to ask for it, a life may depend upon it.

## The Medical History of Depression

References to depression (melancholia) as a medical condition date back to Greece in the fourth century B.C., with the writings of Hippocrates, the "father of medicine." In ancient Greece, melancholy came to be considered an excess of black bile, one of the four humors of the body (blood, black bile, yellow bile, and phlegm) believed to regulate health. As black bile was also considered the driving force in creativity, melancholy had a positive association with the creative temperament. By pointing out the many poets, artists, politicians, Greek heroes, and philosophers, including Plato and Socrates, who were of a melancholic nature, Aristotle perpetuated a positive view of the condition that continued for centuries.[33]

As melancholy began to be viewed as a condition to cure, in the late fourth century, various methods, including bloodletting, were used to eliminate the excess black bile from the body. This approach lasted into the 1800s, when the humoral theory fell out of favor.[34]

In the late 1800s and early 1900s, the German physician Emil Kraepelin studied and documented mental illnesses, providing the foundation for modern psychiatry. Its focus on diagnosis and classification comes from Dr. Kraepelin.[35]

The belief that psychological factors were the cause of depression arose from the work of Sigmund Freud and began to gain cachet in the American medical establishment in the 1920s.[36] The advent of antidepressant medications in the 1950s transformed the psychiatric field, shifting the focus of the causality of mental illness from psychological to biochemical, and turning the profession into a pharmaceutical industry. The idea that psychological factors may contribute to depression has not been completely dismissed, but the small percentage of money devoted to psychotherapeutic treatment in the total amount expended in the treatment of depression shows where the overwhelming emphasis lies.

### The Antidepressant Drug Model

The current conventional medical view is that depression is a brain disorder caused by a deficiency in neurotransmitters, the

11

brain's chemical messengers that enable communication between cells. While there are many different kinds of neurotransmitters, the primary ones involved in the regulation of mood are serotonin, dopamine, epinephrine/norepinephrine, GABA (gamma-aminobutyric acid), and L-glutamate.

Contrary to popular belief, serotonin is not found only in the brain. In fact, only 5 percent of the body's supply is in the brain, with 95 percent distributed throughout the body and involved in many functions.[37]

Serotonin is similarly distributed throughout the brain, where it is "the single largest brain system known."[38] In addition to influencing mood, serotonin is involved in the regulation of sleep and pain, to name but a few of its numerous activities.

Dopamine has a role in controlling sex drive, memory retrieval, and muscles, in addition to mood. GABA operates to stop excess nerve stimulation, thereby exerting a calming effect on the brain. Two important functions of L-glutamate involve memory and the curbing of chronic stress response and excess secretion of the adrenal "stress" hormone cortisol. Epinephrine (also known as adrenaline) and norepinephrine are hormones produced by the adrenal gland. Epinephrine is involved in the stress response and the physiology of fear and anxiety; an excess has been implicated in some anxiety disorders. Norepinephrine is similar to epinephrine and is the form of adrenaline found in the brain;[39] interference with norepinephrine metabolism at certain brain sites has been linked to affective disorders.[40]

Serotonin, dopamine, and norepinephrine are monoamines (they are derived from amino acids) colloquially known as the "feel good" neurotransmitters.[41] As such, they are the target of antidepressant drug action. Prozac, Paxil, Zoloft, Luvox, and Effexor are what is known as SSRIs, selective serotonin re-uptake inhibitors. They block the natural reabsorption of serotonin by brain cells, which boosts the level of available serotonin. SSRIs are relatively new arrivals on the antidepressant scene; Prozac was introduced on the market in 1987.

Earlier categories of antidepressant drugs are tricyclics and monoamine oxidase inhibitors (MAOIs). Tricyclics such as Elavil,

Adapin, and Endep inhibit serotonin re-uptake, but block norepinephrine re-uptake as well; thus, they are less selective than SSRIs. MAOIs such as Nardil and Parnate act by inhibiting a certain MAO enzyme that breaks down monoamines; the outcome is more available neurotransmitters.[42]

The theory that neurotransmitter deficiency causes depression is known as the "biogenic amine" hypothesis. While the model recognizes that imbalances in amino acids (neurotransmitter precursors) produce the deficiency, amino acid supplementation is not the conventional medical solution. "These amino acids have proven to be effective natural antidepressants," states Michael T. Murray, N.D., author of *Natural Alternatives to Prozac.*[43]

Despite this, the focus of conventional treatment is expensive pharmaceuticals. "Perhaps the main reason [the biogenic amine] model is so popular is that it is a better fit for drug therapy," notes Dr. Murray.[44]

Contrary to popular belief, the newer, more expensive antidepressants—Prozac, Zoloft, and Paxil—are no more effective than the older antidepressant drugs, according to a report issued by researchers for the U.S. Agency for Health Care Policy and Research and the U.S. Department of Health and Human Services. Not only that, but research has not established that any drug produces better results than psychotherapy as a treatment for depression, the report reveals.[45]

Antidepressant drugs are problematic for a number of other reasons as well. It is sufficient for the purposes of this book to cite only two. First, the adverse effects (euphemistically known as side effects) of antidepressants can range from uncomfortable to untenable, although some people who take the drugs experience no side effects. With Prozac, for example, adverse effects include nausea, headache, anxiety and nervousness, insomnia, drowsiness, diarrhea, dry mouth, loss of appetite, sweating and tremor, and rash.[46]

Flattened or dulled feelings and sexual dysfunction are common effects of taking SSRIs. In addition, the anxiety and agitation induced by SSRIs can result in patients increasing their use of alcohol and other substances for calming purposes.[47]

More serious, there has been very little research on the long-term effects of taking SSRIs. It is known, however, that they can produce neurological disorders, and permanent brain damage is a danger.[48]

Second, and perhaps most important, antidepressants do nothing to address the deeper causes of depression. Why are the amino acids and neurotransmitters out of balance? What caused that to happen? What are the other factors involved in the depression of this particular individual? Chapter 2 looks at the many causes of depression, which can serve as a starting point for answering these questions.

# 2 Sixteen Causes of Depression

The previous chapter touched upon the notion of mood as an evolutionary adaptation, with depression serving the function of disengaging us from danger, to put it simply. That idea may explain the huge increase in depression that has occurred in the past half-century. Those who were born after 1940 are far more likely to suffer from depression than those who were born prior to that year.[49] The nature of the danger is the question. Is it our toxic world? Is it the level of stress that most of us live under? Is it our modern diet with its attendant nutritional deficiencies? Is it the emotional and spiritual vacuum of the technological age?

It may be that depression is not an adaptation, but rather that all of these factors beleaguer our bodies, minds, and spirits and send us into depression. To recover from depression, we need not know the exact mechanism in operation, but we do need to address the factors that are combining to produce the disorder. This means identifying and treating the imbalances in each individual case of depression because the combination of factors differ and the specifics of each factor vary from person to person.

This chapter looks at 16 causes or contributing factors in depression. While the individual causes may seem to be predominantly physical, psychological, or spiritual in nature, keep in mind that each has reverberating effects on the other levels because body, mind, and spirit are integrally linked.

## Sixteen Causes of Depression

The following factors can produce or contribute to depression:

| | |
|---|---|
| chemical toxicity | neurotransmitter deficiencies or dysfunction |
| heavy metal toxicity | |
| *Candida* overgrowth | medical conditions |
| food allergies | medications |
| intestinal dysbiosis | lack of exercise |
| sensitivity to food additives | lack of light |
| nutritional deficiencies/ imbalances | stress |
| | energy imbalances |
| hormonal imbalances | psychospiritual issues |

## 1. Chemical Toxicity

Toxic overload may be one of the reasons why depression has risen so dramatically in those born after 1940. Humans today are exposed to an unprecedented number of chemicals. Testing of anyone on Earth, no matter how remote the area in which they live, will reveal that they are carrying at least 250 chemical contaminants in their body fat.[50]

The onslaught of chemicals begins in the womb, with the transmission of toxins from the toxic mother to the fetus, and continues with breast-feeding. An infant in the United States or Europe imbibes "the maximum recommended lifetime dose of dioxin" in only six months of nursing. Dioxin, a pesticide by-product, is one of the most toxic substances on Earth.[51] The point is that we start life with an already accumulating toxic load.

In their report, *In Harm's Way—Toxic Threats to Child Development,* the Greater Boston Physicians for Social Responsibility summarize research on lead; mercury; cadmium; manganese; nicotine; pesticides (many of which are commonly used in homes and schools); and solvents used in paint, glue, and cleaning products; dioxin; and PCBs (polychlorinated biphenyls; both PCBs and dioxin stay in the food chain once they enter it, as they pervasively have).

The report notes that in one year alone (1997), industrial plants released more than a billion pounds of these chemicals directly into the environment (air, water, and land). Further, almost 75 percent of the top 20 chemicals (those released in the largest quantities) are known or suspected to be neurotoxicants.[52] (Neurotoxicants are substances that are toxic to the brain and the nervous system in general.) Other sources report that of 70,000 different chemicals being used commercially only 10 percent have been tested for their effect on the nervous system.[53] In addition to the pesticides used directly on crops, the chemicals in the air, water, and soil are fully integrated into our food supply.

Chemical toxicity is known to produce depression. "In the earliest form of chronic toxicity, mild mood disorders predominate as the patient's chief complaint," states an official at the National Institute for Occupational Safety and Health.[54] People who suffer from chemical sensitivity, which is on one end of the continuum of the effects of chemicals on the body, know well the depression that accompanies the condition.

The rest of us who are not yet so overtly sensitive are still absorbing the effects of the toxins in our environment, and those chemicals are exerting their influence on our mood. "Everyday chemicals have the potential to interfere with the metabolism of brain neurotransmitters or happy hormones in a myriad of pathways," says Sherry A. Rogers, M.D., author of *Depression—Cured at Last!* "They interfere with synthesis and metabolism, they block receptor sites, poison enzymes, and much more."[55]

As just one example of how this works, consider the hydrazines, a family of widely used chemicals, notably in pesticides, jet fuels, and growth retardants. Hydrazine is sprayed on potatoes to prolong their shelf life. In the body, this chemical blocks serotonin production by blocking the action of vitamin $B_6$, which is needed at every step in the series of enzyme actions required in the manufacture of serotonin. In just one bag of potato chips or one serving of fast-food French fries, there is sufficient hydrazine to knock out all the B$_6$ in your body.[56]

## 2. Heavy Metal Toxicity

"Historians have theorized that one of the reasons the Roman empire declined was as a result of contamination from lead pipes," writes Catherine Carrigan in *Healing Depression*. "A hundred years from now, future historians may reckon that one of the reasons depression increased so rapidly in our society was as a result of widespread exposure to toxic metals."[57]

Mercury, copper, lead, and aluminum are "the worst culprits" among the heavy metals that can cause depression.[58]

The heavy metal mercury is well-recognized as a neurotoxin, and has been for centuries. Early hatmakers contracted what was known as "mad hatter's disease," the result of poisoning from the mercury used in hatmaking, hence the saying, "mad as a hatter." Physiologically, mercury's effects on the brain arise from its ability to bond firmly with structures in the nervous system, explains Dr. Dietrich Klinghardt, whose work is featured in chapter 3. Research shows that it is taken up in the peripheral nervous system by all nerve endings (in the tongue, lungs, intestines, and connective tissue, for example) and then transported quickly via nerves to the spinal cord and brainstem.

"Once mercury has traveled up the axon, the nerve cell is impaired in its ability to detoxify itself and in its ability to nurture itself," says Dr. Klinghardt. "The cell becomes toxic and dies—or lives in a state of chronic malnutrition. . . . A multitude of illnesses, usually associated with neurological symptoms, result."[59]

Mercury is bioaccumulative, which means that it doesn't break down in the environment or in the body. The result is that it is everywhere in our environment, in our food, air, and water, and each exposure adds to our internal accumulation. Many of us also carry a source of mercury in our mouths in the form of dental fillings; so-called silver fillings are actually comprised of over 50 percent mercury. These fillings leach mercury, predominantly in the form of vapor, 80 percent of which is absorbed through the lungs into the bloodstream. Chewing raises the level of vapor emission and it remains elevated for at least 90 minutes afterward.[60]

Among the symptoms that improve after having mercury amalgam fillings replaced with nontoxic composite fillings are depression, fatigue, lack of energy, anxiety, nervousness, irritability, insomnia, headaches, memory loss, lack of concentration, allergies, gastrointestinal upset, and thyroid problems. In a survey of 762 people conducted by the Foundation for Toxic Free Dentistry of Orlando, Florida, 23.75 percent (181) of the subjects reported that they had suffered from depression prior to having their mercury fillings replaced, and all of them reported that their depression disappeared afterward.[61]

*Depression, fatigue, and headaches, among numerous other symptoms, can result from an intestinal overgrowth of* **Candida albicans,** *the yeast-like fungus normally found in the body. The fungus, through its normal metabolic processes, releases substances that are toxic to the brain and interfere with neurotransmitter activity.*

Copper is also found in dental fillings, often added as an alloy to gold fillings. Other sources of copper exposure are cigarettes, cookware, and water pipes. Lead exposure is often an occupational hazard; approximately one million Americans are exposed to lead on the job.[62] Other sources of exposure include certain glazed ceramics, old paint, water pipes, fertilizers, and soft vinyl products. In 1996, cheap vinyl miniblinds were recalled due to a high lead content. Other products with even higher lead contents are still on the market. For example, one manufacturer's rain suit for children tested at two percent lead, which is almost one hundred times the amount allowed in mini-blinds.[63]

In addition to depression, aluminum toxicity has been linked to Alzheimer's, gastrointestinal problems, and liver dysfunction.[64] Among the common sources of aluminum exposure are cookware, aluminum salts in baking powder, aluminum-containing anta-cids, and many antiperspirants and deodorants.

In chapter 4, Thomas M. Rau, M.D., a pioneer in biological medicine, also discusses the heavy metals palladium and platinum in relationship to depression.

## 3. Candida Overgrowth

Depression, fatigue, and headaches, among numerous other symptoms, can result from an intestinal overgrowth of *Candida albicans,* the yeast-like fungus normally found in the body. There are a dozen different mechanisms by which *Candida* overgrowth produces depression. One is that the fungus, through its normal metabolic processes, releases substances that are toxic to the brain and interfere with neurotransmitter activity.[65]

As noted in the section on intestinal dysbiosis to follow, bac-teria, yeast, and other substances in the intestines can travel to the brain via the bloodstream. Another mechanism by which *Candida* overgrowth produces depression is that the intestinal lin-ing becomes inflamed, which interferes with the absorption of nutrients.[66] As discussed later, nutritional deficiencies are impli-cated in depression.

*Candida* overgrowth occurs when something intervenes to disturb the normal balance of flora in the intestinal environment. The main culprit in throwing off the balance is antibiotics, par-ticularly the repeated use of antibiotics, which kill all the benefi-cial bacteria that keep potentially harmful flora such as *Candida* in check. Weakened immunity may also be a factor in yeast over-growth.

Eliminating foods that "feed" *Candida* is a common treat-ment approach to restoring intestinal balance. The so-called Candida diet emphasizes avoiding all forms and sources of sugar, including fruit and fruit juice, carbohydrates, and fermented yeast products.

A number of natural medicine practitioners, notably Dr. Thomas Rau (see chapter 4) have discovered the connection between *Candida* and mercury, postulating that one of the functions of the fungus in the body is to deal with heavy metals such as mercury, for which it has a particular affinity. If there is a high level of mercury in the body, *Candida* multiplies. Until you detoxify the body of the mercury, says Dr. Rau, you won't be able to get rid of the *Candida* overgrowth on any lasting basis, no matter how perfect your diet or what antifungal drug or natural substance you take. The fungus will just keep coming back.[67]

## 4. Food Allergies

Depression, fatigue, and headaches are the most common symptoms of food allergies in adults. Mood symptoms run the gamut from mild anxiety to serious depression.[68] Many people are not aware that they are suffering from food allergies, as the symptoms are often not clearly linked with ingestion of the food, as is the case when someone breaks out in a rash after eating strawberries or experiences a dangerous constriction of air passages after eating shellfish.

A discussion of allergies involves both what happens in the body on a physical level and the imbalance in the energy field that an allergy entails. The latter is why NAET (Nambudripad's Allergy Elimination Techniques; see chapter 3), which employs acupuncture among other techniques to restore the body's energy flow in relation to the allergen (substance to which one is sensitive or allergic), is effective in eliminating allergies. Disturbances in the flow of energy by themselves produce a range of symptoms, including depression, as is detailed in many of the chapters in part 2.

Seeming allergies may actually be intolerances or sensitivities resulting from compromised immune and digestive systems or energy disturbances. Once these factors are eliminated or eased, the food intolerances may disappear.

Food intolerances occur when the body doesn't digest food adequately, which results in large undigested protein molecules entering the intestines from the stomach. When poor digestion is chronic, these large molecules push through the lining of the intestines, creating the condition known as leaky gut, and enter the bloodstream. There, these substances are out of context, not recognized as food molecules, and so are regarded as foreign invaders.

The immune system sends an antibody (also called an immunoglobulin) to bind with the foreign protein (antigen), a process which produces the chemicals of allergic response. The antigen-antibody combination is known as a circulating immune complex, or CIC. Normally, a CIC is destroyed or removed from the body, but under conditions of weakened immunity, CICs tend to accumulate in the blood, putting the body on allergic alert, if you will. Thereafter, whenever the person eats the food in question, an allergic reaction follows.

It is important to consider here the concept of "brain allergies." Until recently, allergies were thought to affect only the mucous membranes, the respiratory tract, and the skin. A growing body of evidence indicates that an allergy can have profound effects on the brain and, as a result, on behavior. An allergy or intolerance that affects the brain is known as a brain allergy or a cerebral allergy.

The intestinal dysfunction inherent in food allergies itself contributes to depression, as discussed in the next section.

## 5. Intestinal Dysbiosis

Intestinal dysbiosis means an imbalance of the flora that normally inhabit the intestines. Among these flora are the beneficial bacteria (known as probiotics) *Lactobacillus acidophilus* and *Bifidobacterium bifidum,* potentially harmful bacteria such as *E. coli* and *Clostridium,* and the fungus *Candida albicans,* as discussed previously. When the balance among these flora is disturbed, the microorganisms held in check by the beneficial bacteria proliferate and release toxins that compromise intestinal function. This has far-reaching effects in the body and on the mind.

Research has revealed that what passes through the lining of the intestines (see Food Allergies) can make its way through the bloodstream to the brain.[69] As an example of just one of the results of this relationship, in the brain certain intestinal bacteria can interfere with neurotransmitter function.[70] Depression and fatigue are two of the many health problems that can result from intestinal dysbiosis.

Anti-inflammatory drugs, antibiotics, food allergies, and a poor diet are among the factors that contribute to intestinal dysbiosis.

## 6. Sensitivity to Food Additives

Food additives can produce a range of effects from depression, insomnia, nervousness, and hyperactivity to dizziness, blurred vision, and migraines. Research has established that aspartame (an artificial sweetener), aspartic acid (an amino acid in aspartame), glutamic acid (found in flavor enhancers and salt substitutes), and the artificial flavoring MSG (monosodium glutamate) are neurotoxins.[71] Aspartame and MSG are particularly implicated in depression. Depression is one of the frequent complaints to the FDA (Food and Drug Administration) associated with ingestion of aspartame.[72] Aspartame alters amino acid ratios and blocks serotonin production.[73] MSG has been shown to affect serotonin levels.[74]

The more than 3,000 additives used in commercially prepared food have not been tested by their manufacturers for their effects on the nervous system or on behavior.[75] In addition to those mentioned above, common food additives are artificial flavoring, artificial preservatives (BHA, BHT, and TBHQ are in this category), artificial coloring/food dyes, thickeners, moisteners, and artificial sweeteners.

Sensitivity to food additives varies; a high sensitivity may reflect an already large toxic load or weakened immunity. Noticing if your depression worsens after ingesting certain foods

> ## In Their Own Words
>
> *"For 18 years I took the very best pills, followed the advice of countless well-meaning psychiatrists, and spent untold hours talking out the complexities of a difficult life. Despite the amount of money, time, and effort devoted to my mental health, I never knew what it meant to be mentally balanced until I was forced, by ill health, to find this alternative path."*
>
> —Catherine Carrigan, on her recovery from depression[76]

can start the process of elimination for determining which additives, if any, are problematic for you.

## 7. Nutritional Deficiencies and Imbalances

Nutritional deficiencies and imbalances are another common feature of depression. The nutrients most implicated are essential fatty acids, amino acids, the B vitamins, and magnesium.

Again, no two people with depression will have the exact same nutritional condition. Blood chemistry analysis can determine the precise status of your nutrient levels. With this information, therapeutic intervention can then be tailored to your specific nutrient needs. Random supplementation may not address those needs and may even contribute to further skewing of nutrient ratios.

*Essential Fatty Acids:* Research has discovered a link between lipids and mental disorders. Lipids are fats or oils, which are comprised of fatty acids. Examples of saturated fatty acids are animal fats and other fats, such as coconut oil, that are solid at room temperature. Examples of unsaturated fatty acids, which remain liquid at room temperature, are certain plant and fish oils. Essential fatty acids (EFAs) are unsaturated fats required for many metabolic actions in the body.

There are two main types of EFAs: omega 3 and omega 6. The primary omega-3 EFAs are: ALA (alpha-linolenic acid); DHA (docosahexaenoic acid); and EPA (eicosapentaenoic acid). ALA is found in flaxseed and canola oils, pumpkins, walnuts, and soybeans, while DHA and EPA are found in the oils of cold-water fish such as salmon, cod, and mackerel.

Two important types of omega-6 EFAs are GLA (gamma-linolenic acid) and linoleic acid or cis-linoleic acid. Evening primrose, black currant, and borage oils are sources of GLA, while linoleic acid is found in most plants and vegetable oils, notably safflower, corn, peanut, and sesame oils. The body converts omega-3 and omega-6 EFAs into prostaglandins, which are hormone-like substances involved in many metabolic functions, including inflammatory processes.

The ratio of omega-3 to omega-6 EFAs is skewed in the standard American diet, which is deficient in omega 3s. High consumption of hydrogenated oils and beef contributes to the skewed ratio. Hydrogenated oils (which are oils processed to extend shelf life) are detrimental in two ways: not only does refining oil reduce its omega-3 content, but hydrogenated oils also interfere with normal fatty acid metabolism. Hydrogenated oils, also known as trans-fatty acids, are found in margarine, commercial baked goods, crackers, cookies, and other products. The problem with conventionally raised beef cattle is that they are grain-fed rather than grass-fed; grain is high in omega 6 and low in omega 3, while grass provides a more balanced ratio.[77]

Andrew Stoll, M.D., a psychopharmacology researcher and an assistant professor of psychiatry at Harvard Medical School, states: "Omega-3 fatty acids . . . are essential nutrients for human brain development and general health. Over the past 50 to 100 years, there has been an accelerated deficiency of omega-3 fatty acids in most Western countries. There is emerging evidence that this progressive omega-3 deficiency is responsible, at least in part, for the rise in the incidence of heart disease, asthma, major depression, bipolar disorder, and perhaps autism."[78]

Lipids are necessary for the health of the blood vessels that feed the brain and comprise 50 to 60 percent of the brain's solid matter.[79]

More specifically, nerve cells in the brain contain high levels of omega-3 fatty acids.[80]

A deficiency could obviously have serious consequences. There is a large body of research connecting essential fatty acid deficiencies with depression and other mental disorders. The following is just a sampling of the extensive research findings:

• There is a correlation between severity of depression and omega-3 fatty acid levels. The lower the levels, the more severe the depression.[81]

- Low DHA levels have been linked to low brain serotonin levels, which are associated with a greater tendency toward depression, suicide, and violence.[82]

- Low-fat diets, which typically involve a reduced intake of omega-3 and an increased intake of omega-6 EFAs, can increase the risk of depression.[83]

- One study correlated fish consumption and the incidence of major depression per 100 people in nine countries. The countries with the lowest consumption of fish had the highest incidence of depression, and vice versa.[84]

*Amino Acids:* The production of neurotransmitters that regulate mood requires the presence of certain amino acids or precursors. Tryptophan is the amino acid precursor for serotonin; phenylalanine and tyrosine are the precursors for dopamine and norepinephrine.

Amino acids are the basic building blocks of protein. The body does not manufacture most of the amino acids it requires, so they must be obtained through protein in the diet. With a deficient diet, the body is not able to produce sufficient neurotransmitters, and depression can be the result.

As briefly mentioned in chapter 1, amino-acid supplementation can be effective in alleviating depression and serves as a safe and far less expensive alternative to prescription drugs. Although it may not address the root cause of amino-acid deficiency, such as a poor diet, it corrects the problem, unlike antidepressants. It also increases the supply of neurotransmitters naturally, by simply supplying the body with the building materials it needs, instead of forcing the brain and the neurotransmitters into unnatural function to keep the neurotransmitters available.

One study of the effects of tryptophan supplementation was conducted with 11 patients whose depression was so severe that they were hospitalized. After just a month of supplementation, standard psychiatric tests revealed that the overall depressive states of the 11 patients had dropped by 38 percent. In 7 of the 11, guilt, anxiety, weight loss, and insomnia were significantly reduced.[85]

In the body, tryptophan is converted into 5-HTP (5-hydroxy tryptophan) and then into serotonin. A plant extract form of 5-HTP, available as a supplement, can also be used to boost serotonin levels. A Swiss study found that the antidepressant effects of 5-HTP were equal to those of the conventional SSRI Luvox (fluvoxamine), with fewer of the subjects in the 5-HTP group experiencing side effects. (High dosages of 5-HTP may produce nausea, other gastrointestinal distress, and drowsiness.)

There has not been as much research on the use of phenylalanine and tyrosine supplements in the treatment of depression as there has been on tryptophan, probably due to the focus on serotonin as it relates to the disorder. Studies indicate, however, that it can be beneficial.[86]

Another beneficial substance, related to amino acids, is SAMe or SAM (S-adenosyl-methionine). A form of methionine, it is manufactured in the body from that amino acid. SAMe is involved in many metabolic processes, including the production of brain chemicals. People suffering from depression may not produce enough SAMe, which can be another factor in a reduced supply of neurotransmitters. "Based on results from a number of clinical studies, it appears that SAM is perhaps the most effective natural antidepressant," states Michael T. Murray, N.D.[87]

*Vitamins and Minerals:* The most common vitamin deficiencies associated with depression are vitamin $B_6$ (pyridoxine), $B_{12}$ (cobalamin), and folic acid (a member of the vitamin B family), all of which are vital to neurotransmitter function.[88]

William Walsh, Ph.D., chief scientist and biochemical researcher at the Health Research Institute and Pfeiffer Treatment Center in Naperville, Illinois, has found that a genetic pyrrole disorder, which causes severe deficiency in vitamin $B_6$, can be a factor in depression.

"A pyrrole is a basic chemical structure that is used in the formation of heme, which makes blood red. Pyrroles bind with $B_6$ and then with zinc, thus depleting these nutrients," explains Dr.

Walsh. As vitamin $B_6$ is necessary for the synthesis of serotonin, the result is a lack of this important neurotransmitter.[89]

Inositol, another member of the B-complex family, and magnesium, are important for nervous system balance, and deficiencies in these nutrients have also been implicated in depression.[90] Magnesium enhances $B_6$ activity and, taken as a supplement, helps prevent the magnesium deficiency that can result from high doses of $B_6$. Deficiencies in vitamin $B_1$ (thiamin) and vitamin C are additionally associated with depression, according to Nobel prize–winner Linus Pauling.[91] Vitamin $B_1$ is known as the "morale vitamin" due to the effects it exerts on mental state and the nervous system.[92]

Poor diet and malabsorption due to gastrointestinal dysfunction are common causes of nutritional deficiencies. The depleted mineral content of the soil in which crops are grown, which translates into food with a lower mineral content than our forebears enjoyed, is a factor as well. Finally, many lifestyle practices and attributes of modern life deplete us of vitamins and minerals, regardless of how well we eat: stress, smoking, alcohol and caffeine consumption, and exposure to pollution and heavy metals such as the mercury in our dental fillings.

Given these factors, the recommended daily allowance (RDA; purportedly, the amount of individual vitamins and minerals our body requires daily, whether from food or supplements) is likely far below our nutritive needs, in most cases. The RDA standard is based on a group norm for preventing nutritional deficiencies. There are two problems with that. One, individual needs diverge widely and two, the level of deficiency the RDAs are designed to avoid is severe. The systems of the body can begin to be compromised long before that degree of deficiency registers. In other words, if you use the RDAs as your guideline, you could be walking around with moderate nutritional deficiencies.

Increasing your intake of foods that contain the nutrients cited is a good idea if you are prone to depression. The following are dietary sources of these nutrients:

- Folic acid: brewer's yeast, green leafy vegetables, wheat germ, soybeans, legumes, asparagus, broccoli, oranges, sunflower seeds

- Inositol: citrus, nuts, seeds, legumes

- Magnesium: parsnips, tofu, buckwheat, beans, leafy green vegetables, wheat germ, blackstrap molasses, kelp, brewer's yeast, nuts, seeds, bananas, avocado, dairy, seafood

- Vitamin $B_1$: brewer's yeast, wheat germ, sunflower seeds, soybeans, peanuts, liver and other organ meats

- Vitamin $B_6$: brewer's yeast, wheat germ, bananas, seeds, nuts, legumes, avocado, leafy green vegetables, potatoes, cauliflower, chicken, whole grains

- Vitamin $B_{12}$: liver, kidneys, eggs, clams, oysters, fish, dairy

- Vitamin C: green vegetables (particularly broccoli, Brussels sprouts, green peppers, kale, turnip greens, and collards), fruits (particularly guava, persimmons, black currants, strawberries, papaya, and citrus; citrus contains less vitamin C than the other fruits)

## 8. Neurotransmitter Deficiencies or Dysfunction

The role of the neurotransmitters serotonin, dopamine, and norepinephrine in depression is covered in chapter 1. There is ample research to support the theory that problems with these "feel good" brain chemicals can produce depression. The focus is often on supply rather than function, however. A normal level of a given neurotransmitter does not guarantee that the mind and body will receive its benefits. For example, despite high blood levels of the neurotransmitter serotonin, reduced uptake in the brain may mean that the availability of this vital nerve messenger is actually limited.[93]

As discussed in chapter 1, simply attempting to correct neurotransmitter supply or even function does not address the root problem of why the supply is low or the neurotransmitters are not working properly. As you will learn in part 2 of this book, treating the root problems, which range from the physical to the spiritual, often results in the neurotransmitter deficiency or dysfunction self-correcting as the body is restored to its innate ability to heal itself.

## 9. Hormonal Imbalances

Hormones "are probably second only to the chemicals of the brain in shaping how we feel and behave."[94] As hormonal imbalances influence brain chemistry and the nervous system, depression is frequently a corollary symptom.[95] The hormones most often implicated are those released by the thyroid gland, the adrenal glands (cortisol, DHEA, epinephrine, and norepinephrine), and the ovaries and testicles (estrogen, progesterone, and testosterone).

Hypothyroidism (an underactive thyroid) is one of the most common hormonal imbalances underlying depression and is often overlooked as a cause because it can be at a subclinical level and still produce depressive symptoms. The primary symptoms of hypothyroidism are depression and fatigue.

In women, too little estrogen in relation to other hormones tends to produce depression, while too much estrogen in relation to other hormones tends to result in anxiety.[96]

Too little progesterone can also lead to depression; this is often the problem with both premenstrual and postpartum depression.[97]

Testosterone deficiency in both men and women (yes, women have testosterone) can result in depression as well.[98]

Of the adrenal hormones, too little DHEA (dehydroepiandrosterone) or too high levels of the stress hormone cortisol have been linked with depression.[99] As discussed in the previous chapter, epinephrine, or adrenaline, is involved in the stress response and anxiety, while norepinephrine, the form of adrenaline found in the brain, is one of the "feel good" neurotransmitters and as such has influence in affective disorders.

Toxic exposure, stress, diet, and exercise can all affect hormonal levels and balance.

## 10. Medical Conditions

There are a number of medical conditions for which depression is a symptom. Hypothyroidism, as noted above, is one of them. Others include hypoglycemia (low blood sugar), heart disease, lung disease, liver disease, cancer, multiple sclerosis, and rheumatoid arthritis.

## 11. Medications

A wide range of prescription medications can cause depression. Among them are corticosteroids, antihistamines, anti-inflammatories, beta blockers and other antihypertensives, drugs that lower cholesterol, birth control pills, tranquilizers, sedatives, and quinolone antibiotics (Cipro and Floxin).[100]

## 12. Lack of Exercise

Exercise stimulates the release of endorphins, chemicals that lift our mood and reduce our stress level. Research has shown that exercise can alleviate depression. A German study of people with major depression found that exercise (30 minutes of walking daily) reduced their depression in less than the time it typically takes antidepressants to work. Another study of depression in older adults found that exercise was more effective than antidepressants in alleviating the mood disorder.[101]

Exercise also helps flush toxins out of the body. Given the role of toxins in depression, as enumerated earlier, reducing the toxic load you are carrying around is an important antidepressant measure.

## 13. Lack of Light

Lack of light does not only refer to the reduced light of winter that produces the variety of depression known as seasonal

## Optimism as an Antidepressant

Cultivating optimism is a psychological tool against depression. Research shows that optimists are less likely than pessimists to suffer from depression. In addition, they are less likely to contract infectious illnesses and less likely to develop degenerative diseases. They also earn more than three times the money that pessimists do.[103]

Martin Seligman, Ph.D., pioneered work in the cultivation of optimism as a means of counteracting what he calls learned helplessness, which, simply put in regard to depression, is the belief that nothing will make a difference in one's depression. For more information, see Dr. Seligman's book *Learned Optimism: How to Change Your Mind and Your Life* (Pocket Books, 1998).

affective disorder. It refers to a potentially daily, round-the-year factor in depression that stems from the fact that in this technological age so many of us spend the vast majority of our time indoors under artificial light. Studies have demonstrated the link between lack of light and depression.[102]

Lack of light results in lower levels of serotonin. It also contributes to sleep disorders such as insomnia because it interferes with melatonin function. Melatonin, a hormone important in sleep regulation, is manufactured from serotonin. This helps to explain the intimate relationship between depression and sleep problems. The pineal gland, which manufactures melatonin, depends upon the proper cycle of darkness and light to stimulate or inhibit production.

Spending more time outdoors and using full spectrum light bulbs in your indoor environments are steps you can take to ameliorate this factor in depression. For a more focused treatment, light box therapy, in which you are exposed to more intensive light, may help.

## 14. Stress

Chronic stress wreaks havoc on the body, mind, and spirit and creates a vicious circle. On the physical level, stress drains nutrients and lowers immunity. The nutritional deficiencies result in compromised neurochemistry in the brain, which in turn reduces the body's ability to cope with stress. Lowered immunity opens the body to the development of disease, which further reduces stress coping capability. Depression can be an outcome of all of these factors. Stress can also throw off the balance of the energy system of the body, which can lead to depression.

*From the perspective of traditional Chinese medicine, depression is caused by a disturbance in the individual's vital force, or qi, as manifested by disturbed energy flow along the meridians, or energy channels, throughout the body.*

## 15. Energy Imbalances

All of the following chapters detailing comprehensive natural medicine treatments for depression address the issue of energy imbalance in one way or another. From the perspective of traditional Chinese medicine, as one example, depression is caused by a disturbance in the individual's vital force, or *qi,* as manifested by disturbed energy flow along the meridians, or energy channels, throughout the body. A disturbance in the energy field of the individual can cause, and be caused by, psychological and spiritual issues that contribute to the mood disorder. Part 2 explains and explores in depth energy imbalances as a factor in depression.

## 16. Psychospiritual Issues

As noted earlier, psychological/emotional and spiritual components have the capacity to throw the energy system out of balance and vice versa. Depression is one manifestation of such imbalances. Along with depression, mind and spirit issues can produce myriad physical effects throughout the body, which in turn can compound depression.

The contribution of the mind and spirit in depression is fully explored in part 2. For example, chapter 8 examines how early trauma can be stored in the body as cellular memories that keep depression encrypted in the body. Chapter 9 covers the effects of emotional and psychological trauma on energy and the spirit, while chapter 10 looks at the role of spiritual and psychic factors in depression.

The next chapter provides a model that will help you make sense of the various levels of healing and how they relate to each other.

# PART II

# Natural Medicine Treatments for Depression

# 3 A Model for Healing

While many people speak generally of the body-mind-spirit connection, Dietrich Klinghardt, M.D., Ph.D., based in Bellevue, Washington, has developed a detailed paradigm that explains that connection in terms of Five Levels of Healing: the Physical Level, the Electromagnetic Level, the Mental Level, the Intuitive Level, and the Spiritual Level. Dr. Klinghardt is internationally acclaimed for this brilliant and comprehensive model of healing, for his expertise in neural therapy, and for several effective therapeutic techniques he has developed (see "About the Therapies and Techniques" at the end of this chapter). He trains doctors around the world in all of these approaches and is perhaps the person most responsible for bringing neural therapy to the attention of the medical and lay communities.

The Five Levels of Healing model provides a comprehensive way to approach and understand many chronic illnesses, including depression. Health and illness are a reflection of the state of these five levels. Depression, like any health problem, can originate on any of the five levels. A basic principle of Dr. Klinghardt's paradigm is that an interference or imbalance on one level, if untreated, spreads upward or downward to the other levels. Thus, depression can involve multiple levels, sometimes even all five, if the originating imbalance was not correctly addressed.

Another basic principle is that healing interventions can be implemented at any of the levels. Unless upper-level imbalances are addressed, restoring balance at the lower levels will not produce long-lasting effects. This provides an answer to why rebalancing the biochemistry of the brain does not resolve some cases of depression. Treating the chemistry only addresses the Physical Level of illness and healing and leaves the causes at the Intuitive Level, for example, intact. The brain chemistry will soon be thrown off again by the downward cascade of this imbalance.

The Five Levels of Healing model also provides a useful framework for the natural medicine therapies covered in the rest of this book. You will see that they approach depression by identifying and treating disturbances at the different levels. In keeping with the holism of natural medicine, a number of the therapeutic modalities function on several levels. For example, traditional Chinese medicine (chapter 5) works on both the Physical and the Electromagnetic Levels, while Matrix therapy (chapter 8) works on the Electromagnetic and Mental Levels.

The following sections explore the Five Levels of Healing in detail and identify therapies that can remove various interferences at each level.

## The First Level: The Physical Body

The Physical Body includes all the functions on the physical plane, such as the structure and biochemistry of the body. Interference or imbalance at this level can result from an injury or anything that alters the structure, such as accidents, concussions, dental work, or surgery. "Surgery modulates the structure by creating adhesions in the bones and ligaments, which changes the way things act on the Physical Level," says Dr. Klinghardt.

Imbalance at the first level can also result from anything that alters the biochemistry such as poor diet, too much or too little of a nutrient in the diet or in nutritional supplements, or taking the wrong supplements for one's particular biochemistry. Organisms such as bacteria, viruses, and parasites can also change the host's biochemistry. "They all take over the host to some degree and change the host's behavior by modulating its biochemistry," Dr. Klinghardt explains.

"The whole world of toxicity also belongs in the biochemistry," he says. Toxic elements that can alter biochemistry include heavy metals such as mercury, insecticides, pesticides, and other environmental chemicals. Interestingly, heavy metals operate on both the Physical Level and the next level of healing, the Electromagnetic Level. Due to their metallic nature, they can alter the biochemistry by creating electromagnetic disturbances.

All of these factors at the Physical Level—surgery, injury, dental work, nutritional imbalances, microorganisms, heavy metals and other toxins—can play a role in producing symptoms of mental illness, including depression, according to Dr. Klinghardt.

The therapeutic modalities that function at this level are those that address biochemical or structural aspects, from drug and hormone therapies to herbal medicine and nutritional supplements, as well as mechanical therapies such as chiropractic.

## The Second Level: The Electromagnetic Body

The Electromagnetic Body is the body's energetic field. Dr. Klinghardt explains it in terms of the traffic of information in the nervous system. "Eighty percent of the messages go up to the brain [from the body], and eighty percent of the messages go down from the brain [to the body]. The nerve currents moving up and down generate a magnetic field that goes out into space, creating an electromagnetic field around the body that interacts with other fields." Acupuncture meridians (energy channels) and the chakra system are part of the Electromagnetic Body.

A chakra, which means 'wheel' in Sanskrit, is an energy vortex or center in the nonphysical counterpart (energy field) of the body. There are seven major chakras positioned roughly from the base of the spine, with points along the spine, to the crown of the head (see page 133). As with acupuncture meridians, when chakras are blocked, the free flow of energy in the body's field is impeded.

Biophysical stress is a source of disturbance at this level. Biophysical stress is electromagnetic interference from devices that have their own electromagnetic fields, such as electric wall outlets, televisions, microwaves, cell phones, cell phone towers, power lines, and radio stations. These interfere with the electromagnetic system in and around the body.

For example, if you sleep with your head near an electric outlet in the wall, the electromagnetic field from that outlet interferes with your own. An outlet may not even have to be involved. Simply sleeping with your head near a wall in which electric cables run can be sufficient to throw your field off. The brain's blood vessels typically contract in response to the man-made electromagnetic field, leading to decreased blood flow in the brain, says Dr. Klinghardt.

Geopathic stress, or electromagnetic emissions from the Earth, is another source of disturbance. Underground streams and fault lines are a source of these emissions. Again, proximity of your bed to one of these sources—for example, directly over a fault line—can throw your own electromagnetic field out of balance and produce a wide range of symptoms. Simply shifting the position of your bed in the room may remove the problem.

Interference at the second level can cascade down to the Physical Level. The constriction of the blood vessels in the brain in response to biophysical or geopathic stress results in the blood carrying less oxygen and nutrients to the brain. The ensuing deficiencies are a biochemical disturbance, with obvious implications for brain function and mental health. If such deficiencies have their root at the Electromagnetic Level, however, it is important to know that you cannot fix them by taking certain supplements to correct the biochemistry, cautions Dr. Klinghardt.

For example, if an individual has a zinc deficiency, supplementing with zinc may correct the problem if it is merely a biochemical disturbance (a first-level issue). If the restriction of blood flow in the brain as a result of sleeping too close to an electrical outlet (a second-level issue) is behind the deficiency, taking zinc may seem to resolve the problem, but it will return when the person stops taking the supplement. Moving the bed away from the outlet will stop the electromagnetic interference and prevent the recurrence of a zinc deficiency.

Physical trauma or scars can also throw off the second level. "If a scar crosses an acupuncture meridian, it completely alters the energy flow in the system," observes Dr. Klinghardt. An infected tooth or a root canal can accomplish the same. Heavy metal toxicity, from mercury dental fillings and/or environmental metals in the air, water, and food supply, can block the entire electromagnetic system. "We know that the ganglia can be disturbed by a number of things, but toxicity in general is often responsible for throwing off the electromagnetic impulses." Vaccinations can have the same effect. (Ganglia are nerve bundles that are like relay stations for nerve impulses.)

The therapies that address this level of healing are those that correct the distortions of the body's electromagnetic field. Acupuncture and Neural Therapy (see "About the Therapies and Techniques," at the end of the chapter) are two strong modalities for this level. Neural Therapy's injection of local anesthetic in the ganglion breaks up electromagnetic disturbances. You could call the local anesthetic "liquid electricity," says Dr. Klinghardt.

Another therapeutic modality that functions at the second level is Ayurvedic medicine (the traditional medicine of India). As it employs a combination of herbs and energetic interventions, it actually covers the first two levels of healing: the herbs work on the Physical Level, and the energetic aspect on the Electromagnetic Level.

## The Third Level: The Mental Body

The third level is the Mental Level or the Mental Body, also known as the Thought Field. This is where your attitudes, beliefs, and early childhood experiences are. "This is the home of psychology," says Dr. Klinghardt. He explains that the Mental Body is outside the Physical Body, rather than housed in the brain. "Memory, thinking, and the mind are all phenomena outside the Physical Body; they are not happening in the brain. The Mental Body is an energetic field."

Disturbances at this level come from traumatic experiences, which can begin as early as conception. Early trauma, or an unresolved conflict situation, leaves faulty circuitry in the Mental Body, explains Dr. Klinghardt. For example, if at two years old, your parents divorced and your father was not allowed by law to see you, you may have formed the beliefs that your father didn't love you and that it was your fault your parents broke up because you are inherently bad. These damaging beliefs are faulty mental circuitry.

The brain replays traumatic experiences over and over, keeping constant stress signals running through the autonomic nervous system. These disturbances trickle down and affect the Electromagnetic Level of healing, changing nerve function by triggering the constriction of blood vessels, and in turn, affecting the biochemical level in the form of nutritional deficiency.

It may look like a biochemical disturbance, says Dr. Klinghardt, but the cause is much higher up. "Again, this is a situation you cannot treat with lasting results by giving someone supplements, Neural Therapy, or acupuncture." You have to address the third-level interference, the problem in the Mental Body.

Despite what people may conclude from the related names, so-called mental disorders aren't necessarily a function of disturbance in the Mental Body. The cause can be on any of the five levels, iterates Dr. Klinghardt. In fact, in most cases, the third level is not the source. In his experience, most "mental" disorders arise from disturbances on the fourth level. In all cases, the source level must be addressed or a long-term resolution will not be achieved.

Dr. Klinghardt uses Applied Psychoneurobiology, which he developed, and Thought Field Therapy to effect healing at the third level (see "About the Therapies and Techniques"). Among the other therapeutic modalities that work at this level are psychotherapy, hypnotherapy, and homeopathy.

## The Fourth Level: The Intuitive Body

The fourth level is the Intuitive Body. Some people call it the Dream Body. Experience on this level includes dream states, trance states, and ecstasy, as well as states with a negative association such as nightmares, possession, and curses. The Intuitive Body is what Jung called the collective unconscious. "On the fourth level, humans are deeply connected with each other and also with flora, fauna, and the global environment," says Dr. Klinghardt.

The fourth level is the realm of shamanism. Other healers who can work at this level to remove interference are those who practice transpersonal psychology. Stated simply, *transpersonal* refers to an acknowledgment of the phenomena of the fourth level, "the dimension where [people are] affected deeply in themselves by something that isn't of themselves, that is of somebody else. Transpersonal psychology is really a cover-up term for modern shamanism," observes Dr. Klinghardt.

For healing of the Intuitive Body, Dr. Klinghardt uses what is known as Systemic Family Therapy, or Family Systems Therapy. It addresses interference that comes from a previous generation in the family. In this type of interference, he says, "the cause and effect are separated by several generations. It goes over time and space." Rather than a genetic inheritance of a physical weakness, it is an energetic legacy of an injustice with which the family never dealt.

The range of specific issues that can be the source is vast, but it usually involves a family member who was excluded in a previous generation. When the other family members don't go through the deep process of grieving the excluded one, whether the exclusion results from separation, death, alienation, or ostracism, the psychic interference of that exclusion is passed on. Another common systemic factor involves identification with victims of a forebear.

"A member of the family two, three, or four generations later will atone for an injustice," without even knowing who the person involved was or what they did, explains Dr. Klinghardt. For example, a woman murders her husband and is never found out. She marries again and lives a long life. Three generations later, one of her great-grandchildren is born. To atone for the murder, the child self-sacrifices by, for example, developing brain cancer at an early age, being abused or murdered, or starting to take drugs as a teenager and commiting a slow suicide.

"It's a form of self-punishment that anybody can see on the outside, but nobody understands what is wrong with this child—he had loving parents, good nutrition, went to a good school, and look what he's doing now, he's on drugs. But if you look back two or three generations, you'll see exactly why this child is self-sacrificing." Dr. Klinghardt notes that mental illness is "very often an outcome on the systemic level."

Systemic Family Therapy involves tracing the origins of current illness back to a previous generation. For the discovery process, Dr. Klinghardt uses the Systemic Family Therapy developed by German psychoanalyst Bert Hellinger. Sometimes an event is known in a family, sometimes it is not. By questioning a client, Dr. Klinghardt is usually able to discover an event from a previous generation that is a likely source of interference for the client's current condition. If no one knew about a certain event, such as the murder in the example above, there are usually clues in a family that point to those people as a possible source.

For the therapy, the client or a close relative chooses audience members to represent the people in question. In our hypothetical and composite example, they would be the great-grandmother, great-grandfather, and the new husband. These people come together on a stage or central area. They are not told the story, even when the story is known. "They just go up there not knowing anything, and suddenly feel all these feelings and have all these thoughts come up. . . . Very quickly, within a minute or two, they start feeling like the real people in life have felt, or are feeling in their death now, and start interacting with each other in bizarre ways," says Dr. Klinghardt.

The client typically does not participate, but simply observes. "The therapist does careful therapeutic interventions, but there's very little needed usually." The person put up for the murdered husband stands there, with no idea of what happened in the past, but then he falls to the floor. When someone asks, "What happened to you?" he answers, "I've been murdered." It just comes out of his mouth. Then the therapist asks if he wants to say anything to any of the other people. He speaks to his wife and it becomes clear that she was the one who murdered him. They speak back and forth, and "very quickly, there's deep healing that happens between the two," states Dr. Klinghardt. "Usually we relive the pain and the truth that was there . . . It's very, very dramatic . . . Then the therapist does some healing therapeutic intervention with those representatives."

With removal of the interference that was transmitted down the generations, the client's condition is resolved, although the trickle-down effect to the lower levels of healing may need to be addressed. Often, however, healing at the higher level is sufficient. With balance restored at that level, the other levels are then able to correct themselves.

Dr. Klinghardt likens Family Systems Therapy to shamanic work in Africa, in which healing often has to be done from a distance through a representative because of the impracticability of a sick child, for example, traveling 200 miles from the village to see the medicine man. The representative holds a piece of clothing or hair from that child, and the shaman does the healing work on the stranger. "There's a magical effect broadcast back to the child," says Dr. Klinghardt. "The child often gets well. It's the same principle [with Family Systems Therapy]. We call it surrogate healing." He adds that Systemic Family Therapy has become very popular in Europe in the last two years, while it is still relatively new in the United States.

Dr. Klinghardt has developed a variation of this technique that enables the work to happen with just a practitioner and the patient in a regular treatment room. He accomplishes the same end without representatives of the antecedents, using Autonomic Response Testing (ART, a kind of muscle testing; see "About the Therapies and Techniques") to pinpoint what happened and engage in the dialogues that arise in this work.

He gives the example of a 45-year-old woman who had lived daily with asthma since she was two years old. Through ART, in a kind of process of elimination, Dr. Klinghardt learned that physical causes were not the source of the asthma and that it had to do with exclusion of some kind in a previous generation. Further exploration revealed that this woman's mother had lost a younger sibling when she was two years old. In this case, the woman knew of the event, but that was all she knew. ART confirmed the connection between this buried death and the asthma. Dr. Klinghardt stopped the session at this point, instructing his client to find out what she could about this family occurrence and then come back.

The woman's mother was still alive and told her that the baby died shortly after birth, was buried behind the house without a gravestone or other marker on the site, and was never mentioned again in the family. Everyone knew where the child was buried, but there was an unspoken agreement never to speak of her. Not only that, but the next child born was given the same name, as if the one who had died had never existed or, worse, had been replaced.

"This was a violation of a principle of what we know about Systemic Family Therapy, which is that each member that's born into a family has the same and equal right to belong to the family." Exclusion, even in memory, is a form of injustice, and creates interference energy that is transmitted through the generations. Exclusion of a family member in the past is frequently the source of disturbance at the Intuitive Level, according to Dr. Klinghardt.

The client came back for the second session, and Dr. Klinghardt put her into a light trance state. "In that trance state she was able to contact that being, the dead sibling, and say to her, 'I remember you now, I bring you back into my family, I give you a place in my heart, I will never forget you.' Then she cried, and it was a very transformative experience." He observes that this process required very little guidance from him and took only about 20 minutes.

During the session, the woman made a commitment to go back to the house where the child was buried—it was still a family property—and put a gravestone on her grave. After the session, the woman's asthma was clearly better. She rated it at 50 to 60 percent better, and reported later that it stayed that way. "It took her about three months to put up the gravestone, and she said the day after she set up the gravestone for that child, her asthma disappeared completely," relates Dr. Klinghardt. That was eight years ago and the asthma has not returned.

Dr. Klinghardt and others who practice Family Systems Therapy have seen similar connections in cases of mental illness. Chronic depression or anxiety, schizophrenia, bipolar disorder, addiction, hyperactivity in children, aggressive behavior, and autism can all lead back to systemic family issues. In fact, Dr. Klinghardt estimates that "about 70 percent of mental disorders across the board go back to systemic family issues that need to be treated. People try to treat them psychologically, on the third level, and it cannot work. This is not the right level." Similarly, focusing on the biochemistry (as with antidepressants) is not going to fix the problem when the source is at the fourth level.

## The Fifth Level: The Spiritual

The fifth level is the direct relationship of the patient with God, or whatever name you choose for the divine. Interference in this relationship can be caused by early childhood experiences, past life traumas, or enlightenment experiences with a guru or other spiritual teacher. Of the latter, Dr. Klinghardt says, "Some enlightenment experiences actually turn out to be a block. If the experience occurred in context with a guru, the person may become unable to reach there without the guru. The very thing that showed them what to look for becomes an obstacle."

This level requires self-healing when there is separation or interference in a person's connection to the divine. Direct contact with nature is one way to reforge the connection. "True prayer and true meditation work on this level as ways of getting there, but it's a level where there is no possibility of interaction between the healer and the patient," states Dr. Klinghardt. "I always say if anybody tries to be helpful on this level, run as fast as you can." He notes that gurus and other spiritual teachers belong on the fourth level and have a valuable place there, but have no business on the fifth level. If they trespass into that level, they are putting themselves where God should be, says Dr. Klinghardt. "It's very dangerous."

That said, a number of the therapies in this book clear impediments to spiritual connection at other levels, especially the Mental and Intuitive, thus opening the way for individuals to reestablish balance for themselves on the fifth level.

## Operating Principles of the Five Healing Levels

The levels affect each other differently, depending on whether the influence is traveling upward or downward. Both trauma and successful therapeutic intervention at the higher levels

## Natural Medicine and the Five Levels of Healing

The chart below shows on what level the natural medicine therapeutic modalities in this book function.

| THERAPY | LEVEL | CHAPTER |
|---|---|---|
| Anthroposophic medicine | Mental Body<br>Spiritual Body | 4 |
| Applied Psychoneurobiology | Physical Body<br>Electromagnetic Body<br>Mental Body | 3 |
| Biological medicine | Physical Body<br>Electromagnetic Body | 4 |
| CranioSacral therapy | Physical Body<br>Electromagnetic Body | 8 |
| Family Systems Therapy | Intuitive Body | 3 |
| Flower essence therapy | Mental Body | 7 |
| Homeopathy | Mental Body | 6 |
| NAET (allergy elimination) | Electromagnetic Body | 3 |
| Neural Therapy | Electromagnetic Body | 3 |
| Nutritional/dietary therapy | Physical Body | 3, 4 |
| Psychic/Shamanic healing | Intuitive Body | 10 |
| Psychosomatic medicine | Mental Body | 9 |
| Seemorg Matrix Work | Electromagnetic Body<br>Mental Body | 9 |
| SomatoEmotional Release | Electromagnetic Body<br>Mental Body | 8 |
| Thought Field Therapy | Electromagnetic Body<br>Mental Body | 3 |
| Traditional Chinese medicine | Physical Body<br>Electromagnetic Body | 5 |
| Visceral Manipulation | Physical Body<br>Electromagnetic Body | 8 |

have a rapid and deeply penetrating effect on the lower levels, says Dr. Klinghardt. This means that both the cause and the cure at the upper levels spread downward quickly. For example, if a systemic family issue is strongly present at the fourth (Intuitive) level, it will have profound effects on the first three levels. Similarly, resolving that issue can produce rapid changes in the Physical, Electromagnetic, and Mental Bodies. The lower levels may correct on their own, without further remediation.

At the same time, trauma or therapeutic intervention at the lower levels has a very slow and little penetrating effect upwards. When you get a physical injury (the first level), for instance, it will gradually change your electromagnetic field (the second level), altering the energy flow in your body. It's a slow process, however. The same is true for healing. "If you want to heal an injury on the second level, let's say you have a chakra that's blocked, you can do that by giving herbs and vitamins—biochemical interventions—but it will take years," says Dr. Klinghardt. But if you do an intervention on the third or fourth level, it can correct the blocked chakra on the second level immediately, within seconds or minutes, he notes.

## Depression and the Five Levels of Healing

As stated earlier, depression can be the result of interference or disturbance on any of the Five Levels of Healing. In his practice, Dr. Klinghardt has discovered a number of trends, however. First, he says, "Depression is a typical symptom of mercury toxicity. For me, chronic depression is heavy metal toxicity until proven otherwise. Usually, several things come together with depression, but you take the heavy metals out, and everybody improves."

To get the metals out of the body, Dr. Klinghardt relies on a method called oral chelation (see "About the Therapies and Techniques"), using known natural chelators such as cilantro. He sometimes uses intravenous chelation with the amino acid glutathione, which is more aggressive in getting metals out of the brain. Heavy metal toxicity may be producing disturbances at both the Physical and Electromagnetic Levels, as previously noted. If that is the case, detoxification through chelation will directly benefit both levels.

Another treatment that operates on the Physical Level is dietary modification. With depression, Dr. Klinghardt does metabolic typing, a method to determine the optimum diet for an individual based on their particular metabolism. He has found that depression is often treatable through the diet, as proper nutrition can help regulate mood.

As for the second level, "depression is not primarily an electromagnetic phenomenon," Dr. Klinghardt states, but it is important to consider the possibility of a contribution on this level in terms of sleeping location—the proximity of the bed to an electric outlet or positioning over a fault line or underground stream. If the depression is of recent onset, this is a factor to consider. Did the person recently move to a new home or change the position of the bed in the room? If the second level is involved in this way, simply changing the sleeping location can offer significant or complete relief.

> **With mild to moderate depression that arrives in adult life, a "burn-out type of syndrome" is often the cause, according to Dr. Klinghardt. It is interesting to note that the phrase burn-out reflects the electromagnetic short-circuiting involved in this type of depression, which is produced by an overload of environmental stresses.**

Again, biophysical or geopathic stress amplifies the symptoms of heavy metal toxicity, says Dr. Klinghardt. Heavy metals are found mostly in the brain, where they work like antennae, he explains. They pick up the electromagnetic or geopathic interference, which exacerbates depression and other symptoms.

With mild to moderate depression that arrives in adult life, a "burn-out type of syndrome" is often the cause, according to Dr. Klinghardt. It is interesting to note that the phrase burn-out reflects the electromagnetic short-circuiting involved in this type of depression, which is produced by an overload of environmental stresses. A lifestyle of running too fast in combination with our burden of heavy metals and other toxins, electromagnetic stress from radio and television towers, sitting in the car with the computerized dashboard and the electric fields there, the indoor pollution in the car, and other cumulative stresses lead to a kind of burn-out in the brain, which is perceived as depression.

Reduced brain function, as in memory problems, may accompany the mood affliction, says Dr. Klinghardt, adding that "an overwhelming majority of the population" now suffer from this kind of depression. "It's just amazing that nobody talks about that, nobody seems inclined to want to do something about it. It's a loss of zest of life, people not being enthusiastic about things, not voting anymore, not having any interest."

Short of an antidote to modern life, reducing your particular environmental stresses is paramount to alleviating this type of depression.

Depression that involves third-level (Mental Body) factors is quite different. In considering the contribution on this level, Dr. Klinghardt looks for early childhood trauma. "Depression is often a type of posttraumatic stress syndrome. There was a stressful experience that wasn't negotiated properly—a divorce, a death— and it lingers." With chronic severe depression, early childhood trauma plays a big role, he notes. More specifically, with deep-seated depression that is usually treated with serial antidepressants, the trauma typically took place during the preverbal stage of life, which encompasses conception through the second year. (Yes, early childhood trauma can begin in the womb.)

Suicidal depression usually involves the fourth (Intuitive) level and family systems issues. For example, a woman came to Dr. Klinghardt for therapy after her sister killed herself. The sister had tried to kill herself two times before she was successful. All three times were on July Fourth or within a week of that date; the first when she was 23, the second at 28, and the final, unfortunately successful attempt at the age of 31. "With a little research, we found out that her grandmother was murdered by her husband on the Fourth of July, 40 years before then," says Dr. Klinghardt. "She had no idea about the murder."

When there is a certain time of the year that people get an urge to kill themselves (aside from seasonal issues such as the reduced light of winter), he observes, it is usually because something happened in previous generations of the family for which the descendent is trying to atone by killing himself, or by suffering. Family systems therapy is a way of making peace with the ancestors and releasing the need to atone.

## Marta: Chronic Depression Under Long-term Anxiety

The following case history illustrates the relationship between depression and the levels of healing, and how the therapies Dr. Klinghardt uses remove these interferences and resolve even a seemingly intractable condition. This case also illustrates the close relationship between depression and anxiety, and how one can mask the other.

For eight years, Marta had been suffering from severe anxiety. She couldn't bear to be in a group of people and, in fact, her anxiety had progressed to the point that she rarely left her house. She had been on the tranquilizer Xanax for quite some time and was worried about addiction to the medication. But whenever she tried to go off it, her anxiety got much worse. Recently, the Xanax had stopped working for her. She felt trapped; she had to find something else to keep her anxiety at bay, and yet she was afraid to go off the medication.

At this point, Marta sought the help of Dr. Klinghardt. His testing methods revealed that she was mercury toxic and had allergies to soybeans, wheat, and Xanax. It is common for people to develop an allergy to medications they take for a long time, says Dr. Klinghardt. "When you're allergic to something, there are two outcomes: you are miserable when you take it, or you become addicted to it." The latter was the case with Marta and her prescription drug.

To eliminate the mercury toxicity, Dr. Klinghardt started Marta on oral chelation. He notes that even if the source of the problem is on the fourth level, until you get the mercury out, Family Systems Therapy or other methods won't be able to clear the fourth-level interference. The mercury creates a kind of wall that prevents the other therapies from working. With the heavy metals removed, he has found that the psychological intervention can be accomplished in one to three sessions. In Marta's case, it was one, as you will see.

To address the allergies, he used an allergy clearing technique similar to NAET (see "About the Therapies and Techniques") to eliminate Marta's allergy to Xanax. In the case of wheat and soybeans, Marta opted to remove them from her diet. Immediately after the treatment, she started feeling better. She stayed on the Xanax and soon discovered that it worked once more as it had when she first started taking it.

She returned periodically for treatments to clear her other allergies, and then decided she was ready to try to go off the Xanax, although it was still effective. For this, Dr. Klinghardt used Thought Field Therapy. He asked Marta to think about her anxiety in different situations while he used ART to determine which meridians went into a stress state. Then he tapped points on the meridians involved while she again thought about the various situations that raised anxiety in her.

In most cases, it only takes one treatment with TFT to resolve anxiety, says Dr. Klinghardt. "You treat it once and then it's gone forever." In Marta's case, it took two treatments because there was a situation she forgot to include the first time. She came back to get cleared on that one.

Then Dr. Klinghardt had Marta begin cutting down on the Xanax. Although she was no longer allergic to the medication, the drug is physiologically habit-forming, so withdrawal is a problem. To ease withdrawal symptoms, he gave her intravenous vitamin C and B vitamins twice a week for the three weeks of the weaning process. At the end of that period, she was off the drug, and had made the transition without having to endure the withdrawal symptoms that usually attend such a process.

What happened then led to the revelation of the true source of her anxiety. With the anxiety peeled away, an underlying depression emerged. Marta told Dr. Klinghardt that it had always been there, but she had never really focused on it. The anxiety had seemed more pressing, although in reality the depression was crippling her life as well.

Through Family Systems Therapy using ART, Marta connected the depression with her mother's sudden death in a car accident when Marta was 17. The way she dealt with that loss was to "march forward, and try not to look back." Her operating principle became "Mom is gone and I can do this on my own." It was at that point that her anxiety disorder began, with the ongoing depression beneath it.

According to the tenets of Family Systems Therapy, Marta's refusal to grieve her mother's death was a kind of banishment of her mother from the family. It broke their psychic link and created a disturbance in Marta on the Intuitive Level, which manifested as depression. To remove the interference, she needed to reestablish the link with her mother. Using Applied Psychoneurobiology, Dr. Klinghardt induced in Marta the mild hypnotic state that would allow her to go to the psychic level and reforge the link to her mother. Through this process, Marta was able to recognize that her mother was always with her. After this experience, the depression disappeared and did not return.

## About the Therapies and Techniques

*Applied Psychoneurobiology (APN):* This therapeutic technique was developed by Dr. Klinghardt. Employing his muscle testing method (see ART, following) as a guide, APN uses stress signals in the autonomic nervous system to communicate with a patient's unconscious mind. "You can establish a code with the unconscious mind for yes and no in answer to questions," he explains. "The code is the strength or the weakness of a test muscle." APN can lead the way to the beliefs that underlie illness such as depression, and exchange those beliefs with ones that promote balance in the Mental Body. This can produce dramatic shifts in the health and well-being of the person, notes Dr. Klinghardt.

*Autonomic Response Testing (ART):* ART, also called neural kinesiology, is a system of testing developed by Dr. Klinghardt. It employs a variety of methods, including muscle response testing and arm length testing, to measure changes in the autonomic nervous system. (The autonomic nervous system controls the automatic processes of the body such as respiration, heart rate, digestion, and response to stress.) ART is used to identify distress in the body and determine optimum treatment. In general, a strong arm (or finger, depending on the kind of muscle testing) or an even arm length (in arm length testing) indicates that the system is not in distress. A weak muscle or uneven arm length indicates the presence of a factor that is causing stress to the client's organism.

*Chelation:* This is a therapy that removes heavy metals from the body, among other therapeutic functions. DMPS (2,3-dimercaptopropane-1-sulfonate) is a substance used as a chelating agent, which means that it binds with heavy metals, notably mercury, and is then excreted from the body. DMPS can be administered orally, intravenously, or intramuscularly. Other chelation agents are cilantro, chlorella, alpha lipoic acid, and glutathione.

*NAET (Nambudripad's Allergy Elimination Techniques):* NAET, developed by Devi S. Nambudripad, M.D., D.C., L.Ac., Ph.D., is a noninvasive and painless method for both identifying and eliminating allergies. It uses kinesiology's muscle response testing to identify allergies. Chiropractic and acupuncture techniques are then implemented to remove the energy blockages in the body that underlie allergies, and to reprogram the brain and nervous system not to respond allergically to previously problem substances.

*Neural Therapy:* Developed by German physicians in 1925, neural therapy employs the injection of local anesthetics such as procaine into specific sites in the body to clear interferences in the flow of electrical energy and restore proper nerve function. The interferences, or "interference fields," as they are known in the profession, can be the result of a scar, other old injury, physical trauma, or dental conditions such as root-canaled or impacted teeth, all of which have their own energy fields that can disrupt the body's normal energy flow. Disruption in the body's energy field has far-flung effects, and can manifest in seemingly unrelated conditions. "Any part of the body that has been traumatized or ill—no matter where it is located—can become an interference field which may cause disturbance anywhere in the body," states Dr.

Klinghardt.[104] Neural Therapy injections may be into glands, acupuncture points, or ganglia (nerve bundles that are like relay stations for nerve impulses), as well as scars or sites of trauma.

*Thought Field Therapy (TFT):* Psychotherapist Roger J. Callahan, Ph.D., developed TFT in response to his frustration at the failure of psychotherapy to help certain clients. It combines principles of acupuncture and psychology to heal the Mental Body. It actually operates on the boundary between the second and third levels, the Electromagnetic and the Mental Bodies, says Dr. Klinghardt. "The thought field is like a net that's attached on the outside of the electromagnetic field. Through early childhood trauma, the net is torn off the electric field." TFT restores the attachment points between the electromagnetic and mental fields and restores the proper energy flow in the body's meridians. It accomplishes this through tapping on certain points on the skin. These are acupuncture points that also correspond to the attachment sites, which are slightly out from the body. The tapping functions similarly to the needles in acupuncture, which remove energy blockages and restore the flow of energy along the meridians.

 **Resources** For more information about the therapies or to locate a practitioner near you, see the following:

- *APN, ART, and Neural Therapy:* Dr. Klinghardt (see appendix B); websites: www.neuraltherapy.com and www.pnf.org/neural_kinesiology.html.

- *Chelation:* The American College for Advancement in Medicine (ACAM), 23121 Verdugo Drive, Suite 204, Laguna Hills, CA 92653; fax: 949-455-9679; website: www.acam.org.

- *NAET:* Devi S. Nambudripad, M.D., D.C., L.Ac., Ph.D., Pain Clinic, 6714 Beach Boulevard, Buena Park, CA 90621; tel: 714-523-8900; website: www.naet.com; also see her book *Say Good-Bye to Illness* (Buena Park, CA: Delta Publishing, 1999).

- *TFT: Tapping the Healer Within,* by Roger J.

Callahan, Ph.D. (Chicago: Contemporary Books, 2001); for a practitioner, contact the Callahan Techniques office, 78-816 Via Carmel, La Quinta, CA 92253; tel: 760-360-7832; website: www.tftrx.com (professional site), www.selfhelpuniv.com (self-help site).

# 4 Healing from a Cellular to a Spiritual Level: Biological Medicine

"In most cases, depression is not a psychological problem," states Thomas M. Rau, M.D., a pioneer of European biological medicine and director for the past ten years of the Paracelsus Klinik in Lustmühle, Switzerland, which is dedicated to the practice of biological medicine and dentistry.[105]

Dr. Rau originally trained in and practiced conventional medicine, but grew increasingly frustrated with the poor results that medicine produced in his patients. "I decided that to heal these patients, I must change my medical thinking and try other approaches. I learned my holistic, biological approach slowly, step by step," says Dr. Rau.[106]

Now, in addition to treating patients who come to his clinic from all over the world, he travels extensively to teach biological medicine to other physicians.

"Depression is primarily a liver problem," continues Dr. Rau. By this he means that the liver is deficient in life force, or vital energy. As the liver is the main organ in the body's detoxification system, weakened liver function results in a buildup of toxins in the body, which has a negative effect on the brain and on mood. Neurotoxicity (nervous system toxicity) is known to interfere with the function of neurotransmitters.

**For more about neurotransmitters, see chapter 1 and 2.**

In Dr. Rau's experience, depression is relatively easy to treat. Remove the sources of the liver's depleted energy, "upbuild" the liver, detoxify the body, and depression often resolves itself, he observes. As psychological or spiritual issues can be a cause of liver depletion, however, it's important to address these areas in order to prevent a recurrence of the liver problem and the accompanying depression. This analysis arises from the model of biological medicine.

## What Is Biological Medicine?

Biological medicine is based on the principle that illness is a reflection of imbalance in the body, and imbalance in one part affects the whole. Multiple factors, such as diet; psychological stress; toxic exposure to heavy metals, chemicals, or radiation (or the overuse of pharmaceuticals); intestinal disturbances; and immune system overload; can disturb the natural balance in the body. Thus far, biological medicine is similar to other holistic medical approaches.

What distinguishes biological medicine from these other approaches is that biological medicine identifies disturbances in the natural balance of the body down to the tissue and cellular level, where dysfunctional patterns can be seen (often before they manifest in symptoms). In other words, these multiple factors can throw your cellular function out of whack, which in turn generates the symptoms of illness if balance is not restored. The disturbances in cellular, tissue, and organ function can be identified and remedied. Since cellular function is at the root of all action in the body, restoring balance at the cellular and connective tissue level restores the balance of all body systems and helps the body improve its regulatory functions and its natural ability to heal itself. Thus, looking at the biological (cellular and tissue) terrain of the body, the "internal milieu" as it is known in biological medicine, goes to the roots of illness.

Biological medicine relies on a variety of methods to assess the internal milieu. These include biological terrain assessment, darkfield microscopy, computerized thermography, and heart rate variability. Biological terrain assessment, or BTA, analyzes the blood, urine, and saliva. Among the parameters of the test, the pH levels of all three of these body fluids offer vital clues to the state of the internal milieu. The term pH stands for *potential hydrogen*, and refers to the acid or alkaline (also known as base) level of a solution. If the balance of acidity and alkalinity (the pH balance) is skewed in cells, their function is compromised. Restoring the slightly alkaline state of the body optimizes function and creates an environment inhospitable to disease, which thrives in an acid environment.

Darkfield microscopy involves a specially designed microscope for live blood analysis, which means examination of blood that has just been drawn. (The vials of blood sent to a laboratory in standard blood analysis do not contain live blood. Once outside the body, blood cells generally begin to disintegrate in 10 minutes to 24 hours, depending on conditions.) The examination of live blood offers a distinct set of information not available through a standard blood panel. The appearance of cells, activity between cells, and the presence or absence of foreign microorganisms in live blood provide information on blood cell health, immune activity, and potential disease factors.

Computerized thermography determines how well tissues and organs are functioning by analyzing the temperature at 68 points on the body under different conditions. For example, thermography can show that a person with rheumatoid arthritis has bowel fermentation, food allergies, less than optimal thyroid and kidney function, and chronic sinus inflammation. All of these can be hidden "foci" (sites of interference) that contribute to the picture of illness.

Heart rate variability is a device that tests how well the autonomic nervous system (ANS) is working. The ANS runs the heart, respiration, and digestion, among other vital operations, and also regulates cellular traffic (the flow of nutrients into and toxins out of cells). Problems in ANS function obviously have far-reaching effects, down to the cellular level. Correcting these problems is essential to healing.

## Healing from a Cellular to a Spiritual Level: Biological Medicine

Biological medicine draws from a wide range of therapeutic modalities to restore the chemistry and internal balance of the body. A biological medicine physician may employ dietary changes, nutritional supplements, enzyme therapy, detoxification techniques, phytotherapy (herbal medicine), anthroposophic medicine, acupuncture/traditional Chinese medicine, neural therapy, Cranio Sacral therapy, heat treatments, and/or homeopathy. The latter may consist of: classical homeopathy; combination formulas; drainage remedies that improve organ and tissue capacity to drain toxicities from the body; or preparations called Sanum remedies, which are formulas developed by Dr. Guenther Enderlein, a German bacteriologist and microbiologist whose work in the early decades of the twentieth century became a cornerstone of biological medicine.

Detoxification is another important component of biological medicine treatment. If the body is overloaded with toxins, cellular integrity is compromised and the dysfunction of organs and systems will follow if the load is not reduced. Many diseases, including cancer, are diseases of toxicity.

Finally, biological dentistry is a vital facet of biological medicine. Dental factors, such as mercury toxicity from fillings, root canals, and chronic asymptomatic jawbone infections, are primary causes of disturbance in the body. Biological dentistry recognizes that problems in the teeth can create problems throughout the body, both through blockage of energy and the spread of infection. Correcting teeth and jaw problems is therefore essential in restoring health.

As a holistic medicine, biological medicine regards psychological and spiritual factors as important as physical factors in the creation of illness and the restoration of health. Thus, psychological and spiritual counseling are often part of biological medicine treatment, as is anthroposophic medicine. Anthroposophic medicine, developed in the 1920s by Austrian scientist Rudolf Steiner, is based upon the view that humans are spiritual beings and the body cannot be treated separately from the spirit. The medicines, which are an extension of homeopathic remedies, address the spiritual aspect of a patient. Anthroposophic medicine is widely practiced in Europe, and the number of practitioners in the United States is increasing.

Biological medicine originated in Europe, arising from Dr. Enderlein's theory of pleomorphism, which is in direct opposition to the germ theory advanced by Louis Pasteur in the late 1800s and embraced by conventional Western medicine. In contrast to the view held by the germ theory that bacteria and other microorganisims invade us from without to cause illness, pleomorphism holds that these microbes already exist in us. It is when they change shape (morph), moving through many (pleo) shapes, due to biochemical alterations in the internal milieu of the body, that they produce disease.

Good health depends upon our coexisting in harmony with the millions of microorganisms in our bodies (a state called symbiosis). The toxicities and stress of modern life, and attendant deficiencies, disturb this balance (dysbiosis) and lead to illness if the imbalance is allowed to continue. With pleomorphism as its base, the emphasis in biological medicine is on monitoring the cellular terrain and maintaining or restoring its balance to both prevent and reverse illness.

Some practitioners in the United States are now using the term biological medicine to describe a range of holistic therapies, which may not reflect the mission and focus of the biological medicine that originated in Europe. Those who are rooted in the European tradition of biological medicine, with its focus on cellular terrain, the internal milieu, and the other principles just delineated, use the term European biological medicine to designate that alliance and practice.

 **For information about and referral to practitioners of biological medicine, contact the Biological Medicine Network, c/o Marion Foundation, 3 Barnabas Road, Marion, MA 02738; tel: 508-748-0816; E-mail: bmn@marionfoundation.org.**

## The Liver and Etheric Forces

Stated in simplistic physical terms, the components of depression can be seen as a weak liver and a weak detoxification system. But what causes the weakness? In the anthroposophical view, a deficiency in the liver reflects a deep lack of what Rudolf Steiner called "etheric forces." These are the life forces responsible for building, rebuilding, upbuilding—the vital force that enables the body to build cells, to repair, to replicate, explains Dr. Rau. Yes, the body needs the mechanistic components of proteins and other vital nutrients in order to accomplish this work, but the life force that impels the building is the etheric force, or "etheric body," as it is also termed.

"Depression is very common today because life forces are systematically destroyed," Dr. Rau states. How does this happen? Our toxic world, stress, an overloaded sympathetic nervous system, dental conditions, and psychospiritual factors can all deplete the etheric body.

The stress of modern life has our sympathetic nervous systems running in overdrive. The sympathetic nervous system is one of the two branches of the autonomic nervous system (ANS), which controls the automatic processes of the body such as respiration, heart rate, digestion, and the stress response. In general, the sympathetic branch is associated with arousal and expenditure of body energy; it is the branch involved in the body's mobilization in the face of stress. The second branch, known as the parasympathetic nervous system, in general is associated with a slowing down and a conserving of body energy.

The forces involved in cerebral activity and the sympathetic nervous system are "astral forces," in Steiner's parlance. These are the forces of the ego, the structuring forces that bring thinking and intellectuality into the mass of cells that is the human being, Dr. Rau explains. Modern life involves "too much emphasis on intellectual activities so that the sympathetic nervous system is overactive," he says. "Communicating, thinking, reading . . . these are all intellectual activities that do not fortify etheric forces, and even weaken them." By living your life with a lot of stress and in a cerebrally oriented way, you throw off the natural balance between your etheric and astral forces.

In general, according to Steiner, etheric forces are diminished in someone who is sick. When it comes specifically to depression, such patients have an overload of astral forces and a lack of etheric forces, explains Dr. Rau. "That's why they get like a stone—lack of life energy. And that lack of life energy is reflected in the liver."

It is interesting that the lack of life force is apparent when you look at the blood of a depressed person in darkfield microscopy (see "What Is Biological Medicine?"). "You don't see anything bad on the cells," says Dr. Rau. "They look okay. But the plasma (the protein in the blood that normally moves rapidly) in these patients looks rigid. *Anti-plasma,* we say, meaning it just doesn't look like it has any life in it. Normally, the plasma is much more animated."

In addition to stress and sympathetic nervous system overdrive, your etheric body can also be thrown out of balance by toxins such as heavy metals. This is another chicken-and-egg situation, however. Was your liver weakened by a depletion of your life force, or by toxic overload, which in turn depleted your liver and your life force? In either case, detoxifying the body of the heavy metals is important because failing to do so leaves the burden on the liver intact.

Another source of disturbance of the liver and etheric forces may be found in the teeth in the form of mercury fillings that add to the body's toxic load or problems in the teeth that lie on the same acupuncture meridian (energy channel) that supplies the liver, as you will see in the cases to follow. The "liver teeth" are the eyeteeth or canine cuspids, which are one tooth away from the front teeth on either side. Problems in one or the other of these two cuspids can create an energy disturbance on the Liver acupuncture meridian, which in turn results in an imbalance in the energy supply to the liver, says Dr. Rau.

He often discovers a liver tooth involvement in people who suffer from depression, he notes. The involvement of the teeth in problems throughout the body is why dentistry is an integral part of biological medicine. "All people at Paracelsus with chronic disease, even psychiatric disorders, get a panoramic X ray of their teeth."

*See Also* For more about acupuncture meridians, see chapter 5.

## More about Toxicity

"Most depressive patients are highly toxic," says Dr. Rau. "I have patients who were given the diagnosis of endogenous depression in psychiatric clinics and they were nothing else than mercury toxic." The most common toxic culprits in depression are the heavy metals palladium, lead, mercury, and platinum, he notes. The source of palladium is gold dental fillings. Sources for lead are certain ceramics, paint, water pipes, and fertilizers. Mercury is omnipresent in the environment; food fish and "silver" dental fillings are two of the more specific sources. Platinum comes to humans from unleaded gasoline, which requires it as a catalyst. Dr. Rau notes that the platinum concentration is extremely high in people who live in countries, such as the United States, where unleaded fuel is the norm.

In addition to heavy metals, another source of toxicity Dr. Rau has often found in depression is intestinal dysbiosis. In dysbiosis, the balance of intestinal flora is skewed; that is, the beneficial bacteria that normally populate the intestines are not sufficient in number to keep harmful bacteria in check.

Dysbiosis contributes to a buildup of toxins in the body in two ways. One, the harmful bacteria's normal metabolism processes release toxic by-products. Two, a compromised intestinal system cannot adequately filter toxins, which is one of the important functions of the intestinal lining. Normally, bile from the liver goes through the intestines where toxins are filtered out, and the bile is then recirculated, cleansed. When the intestines are not working correctly, bile is returned to the body with

*The lack of life force is apparent when you look at the blood of a depressed person in darkfield microscopy. "You don't see anything bad on the cells," says Dr. Rau. "They look okay. But the plasma (the protein in the blood that normally moves rapidly) in these patients looks rigid. It just doesn't look like it has any life in it. Normally, the plasma is much more animated."*

the old toxicity, Dr. Rau explains. This condition is known as enterohepatic toxicity (*entero* for intestines and *hepatic* for liver).

An overgrowth of the *Candida* fungus in the intestines also contributes to enterohepatic toxicity. Mercury is often implicated in this overgrowth because "the purpose of *Candida* in the human being is to protect the body from mercury by absorbing it," says Dr. Rau. The mechanism was never intended, however, to deal with large amounts of mercury. Nevertheless, when mercury levels in the body are high, the population of *Candida* multiplies in a vain attempt to deal with the heavy metal load.

### Psychospiritual Factors

Different factors combine to produce depression in different individuals, notes Dr. Rau. The question of why some people with enterohepatic toxicity do not develop depression while others become depressive or schizophrenic can be answered by considering psychospiritual factors and/or a constitutional tendency or a tendency based on familial behavioral models, he says.

"If you have a toxicity and a tendency for depression, then another load comes, for example, a spiritual load, you get depressive." That spiritual load may be a loss of a sense of meaning, whether as the result of a traumatic life event or other cause. The loss of purpose or meaning has reverberations not only in the spirit, but throughout the mind and body as well. That spiritual load may be what tips the etheric body and the liver into energy depletion.

## Biological Medicine Treatment of Depression

Biological medicine begins by identifying what is happening in the body on a cellular level via testing methods discussed earlier. Dr. Rau takes exception to the so-called natural approach to depression and other illness that simply involves the substitution of an herb or other natural medicine for a prescription antidepressant or other medication. This is "still thinking like conventional medicine," he says, regardless of the medicine used. A comprehensive and accurate approach to treatment is to determine exactly what is occurring in the cellular terrain, and then to begin there "to clean and to build up the milieu."

Testing in cases of depression often reveals that the liver energy is indeed depleted. In these cases, treating depression becomes a matter of upbuilding the etheric forces. This is accomplished through dietary changes, detoxification and support of the liver and intestines, restoration of the intestinal milieu, and the administration of Enderlein remedies and anthroposophic remedies, which address the specific body, mind, and spirit factors present in the individual. Any dental involvement is also resolved.

In terms of therapeutic measures to upbuild the liver, Dr. Rau inserts a word of caution for those patients whose depression is acccompanied by suicidal impulses. Upbuilding the life force energy too quickly, when other components of the depression have not been adequately addressed, can result in the person acting on the suicidal impulses as he or she suddenly has more physical energy.

Dr. Rau's general dietary recommendations for someone whose liver is compromised is to avoid animal protein because processing it adds to the liver's load. A vegetarian diet is easier on the liver. Dr. Rau also advises his patients to eliminate dairy products from their diet because dairy tends to congest the lymph system, which is another important part of the body's detoxification system. In addition, many people are allergic or sensitive to dairy, which adds to congestion. Depression reflects a lack of movement in the body, so anything that contributes to congestion is to be avoided.

Certain supplements may be needed to correct nutritional deficiencies that tend to be present with lower metabolic function in the liver. "The copper level is often elevated in depressive patients," Dr. Rau observes. This is evident in hair analysis and in blood (serum) tests. "It's a sign of liver toxicity, a sign of metabolic pathways that are blocked." With high copper comes low zinc because the two operate in ratio to each other. Zinc is needed for many enzymatic processes, including liver metabolism, so the consequences of low zinc are clear. As a supplement, "zinc is generally good for all mental diseases," says Dr. Rau. When copper is high, the trace element lithium is also low in the body. For that reason, it is often necessary to supplement with a natural form of lithium as well as zinc.

Many natural medicine physicians have found that the B vitamins are very effective in ameliorating depression. This makes sense, as depression is a lack of energy, and the B vitamins are "energy" vitamins. More specifically, Dr. Rau uses B complex, with a focus on $B_6$ and $B_{12}$, to activate the liver.

Dr. Rau generally uses the classic plant remedies for activating and supporting the liver: dandelion (*Taraxacum officinalis*), milk thistle (*Carduus marianus*), and wormwood (*Artemisia absinthum*). If the cellular terrain is clear, then these herbs are not necessary. In that case, Dr. Rau may turn to homeopathy to address the emotional and psychological aspects of the depression. His modus operandi is to stabilize the patient first, meaning restore the cellular terrain and get everything working well on the physical level. "My experience is that if you clean the patient's milieu, afterwards pure homeopathy works much better."

*See Also* For more about homeopathy, see chapter 6.

In most cases, Dr. Rau reports, this program, tailored to the individual's specific cellular terrain status, is effective and other measures are not required. With the sources of toxicity and etheric depletion removed, the patient's neurotransmitter dysfunction corrects itself and the depression is resolved.

## From Dr. Rau's Case Files

Greta, 25, was severely depressed and had been for three years. A psychiatric hospital had diagnosed her with psychotic depression. She was suicidal and on antidepressants. She didn't come to Dr. Rau for treatment of her depression, however, because she had given up hope in that arena. She had severe acne, also of three years standing, and had heard that he might be able to help.

Greta's was "a classical toxic depression case," says Dr. Rau. Testing revealed one of the highest levels of mercury that he had ever seen. In addition to its contribution to depression, mercury can cause skin disease, he notes. Greta had numerous mercury dental fillings as well as four impacted wisdom teeth. The latter were "an expression of long-term emotional problems," observes Dr. Rau, an indication of a lack of development of the self, what he calls a sense of "I am I."

Although she eventually had her wisdom teeth pulled, the pivotal treatments in her case were having her mercury fillings replaced with non-mercury composite fillings and undergoing detoxification via homeopathic drainage remedies. These resolved both her depression and her acne. She was able to get off the antidepressants and has now been free of depression for two years.

Obviously, mercury was a primary cause in Greta's depression, but it is impossible to say what factors tipped the balance for her. Perhaps the mercury overload on top of the psychological factor of a lack of a sense of self brought the depletion of her etheric body to the point that it produced depression.

Danielle, 40, also suffered from psychotic depression and was on antidepressants. Ironically, she was a high-level employee in a natural medicine product company. She had been unable, however, to find a solution to her debilitating depression. When she

> ## Sanum Remedies
>
> Sanum remedies are isopathic formulas developed by Dr. Gunther Enderlein to restore the milieu of the body (see "What Is Biological Medicine?"). The term isopathic is more accurate in describing the remedies than the term homeopathic. *Iso* means "equal," whereas *homeo* means "like." Sanum remedies are actually derived from microorganisms or protein particles, whereas homeopathic remedies are derived from substances that produce symptoms in a healthy person similar to a certain disease condition. Sanum remedies restore the cellular terrain to a healthy state and stimulate the pathogenic microorganisms to revert to their harmless forms. Sanum remedies are available only through health practitioners.

came to Dr. Rau and he ordered the standard dental X ray, she said, "I have beautiful teeth. Why are you x-raying them?" He explained the connection between the teeth and the rest of the body via the acupuncture meridians.

She was further enlightened when the X ray showed that she had an impacted tooth in the liver tooth area on one side. Dr. Rau describes the significance of this as "retracted liver energy," which was fine as long as she was a child, but it meant she "couldn't do adult energy." The result of the energy deficiency was that as an adult she saw the world as grey.

Removing the impacted tooth was enough to begin to restore color to her world. Slowly, her etheric, liver energy rebuilt itself and she grew more interested in life. Now, five years later, she is full of energy and considered "the pearl" of her company.

Fritz, 45, was the manager in a company of 40 employees. He suddenly began having problems with anger at work, blowing up at his employees for no reason. He alternated between this and negativity and a lack of interest in anything around him. He had consulted a doctor who labeled his condition depression and put him on antidepressants.

"Every morning I'm afraid of going to work because I know it could happen from nothing that I explode and shout at my people. And if it continues this way, they won't stand for it anymore," Fritz told Dr. Rau.

Fritz was also having trouble sleeping, from worry over his behavior and an inability to calm down. He had begun drinking quite a bit of wine at night so he could fall asleep.

Exploding followed by negativity are classic signs of liver imbalance, as is difficulty sleeping, says Dr. Rau. Dental X rays identified a source of the problem, showing osteopenia (bone loss) in one of the liver teeth. The gum was retracted and the bone around the tooth was weak. There was no infection, only atrophy.

Neural therapy (using injections of the local anesthetic lidocaine and anthroposophic remedies for the liver) on the apex of the tooth removed the energy interference that the osteopenia was producing on the liver acupuncture meridian and helped upbuild the depleted liver. The latter was also accomplished with high doses of vitamin B, an Ayurvedic liver remedy called Liv 52, and the Sanum remedy Mucedokehl, which balances the liver milieu and works well with emotional-mental conditions. This treatment was effective and Fritz was soon no longer depressed, angry, or explosive.

*See Also* **For more about neural therapy, see chapter 3.**

In most of Dr. Rau's depression cases, as with the three patients already mentioned, there is no need to progress to addressing psychospiritual components. "That doesn't mean there are no mental or spiritual factors in depression," states Dr. Rau, "but that it's important to look at functional causes."

## More about the Spirit

Bradford S. Weeks, M.D., whose practice is based in Clinton, Washington, is another doctor who is highly skilled in biological medicine, with a focus on anthroposophic medicine. Like Dr. Rau, he originally trained in conventional medicine, in two particularly rigorous fields of study—neurology and psychiatry. Now his practice (and the workshops, seminars, and lectures he regularly delivers) is devoted to addressing the body, mind, and spirit components of illness—in other words, to treating his patients holistically. "In my opinion, everybody coming in is a psychiatric patient," Dr. Weeks notes. "By this I mean that everyone has compounding spiritual issues that affect the soul and the physical body. I don't make a distinction between psychiatric illnesses and other illnesses."

Like Dr. Rau, however, Dr. Weeks attends to the physical and etheric processes first, addressing biochemistry, toxicity, life force, natural rhythms, and sleep disruption. Dr. Weeks tells his patients, "You've got a physical body. We have to address the biochemistry. But you also have a soul. You have to feed the soul. Then there's the spirit."

He explains to them that the health of their soul requires that they learn how to nurture themselves. "You've got to have ice cream sometimes, or you've got to go for a walk, or you've got to tell your boss off, or you've got to create some space and take care of yourself. So many people are pathologic caregivers. That's why far more women are depressed than men." Part of the work that Dr. Weeks does is to get people thinking about and starting to develop ways to nurture themselves.

In considering the emotional and psychological factors in depression, Dr. Weeks analyzes it in this way: "What happens with depression is people get sad for a while, and nobody really cares, so they start to become mad or angry. After they become mad or angry and nobody really cares, they start to do bad things like shooting up a post office. Everyone who is mad is fundamentally sad." With that in mind, the productive line of inquiry is not "Tell me about your anger," but rather, "Why are you sad?"

Another aspect of exploring the psychological dimension is helping people to see that they are partly responsible for allowing themselves to be depressed, according to Dr. Weeks. "If they don't buy it, I'll say, 'Well, you're feeling depressed, right? How do you think you'd feel if you watched your daughter walk out into traffic, and you saw a car approaching? Guess what? The depression disappears because the dominant thought is now fear and concern for your child's safety.'" The point he is making to his patients is that we are all in a position to determine what we think about. "People need to appreciate the fact that they're responsible for their reality. Their reality is entirely dependent upon their thought process."

He emphasizes that this does not translate into blaming people for having depression. It is a matter of information and understanding. Dr. Weeks tries to help his patients to see that they have control over what they choose to think about. "'Yes, your mother was a mean mother to you. I'm sorry that happened. I'm sorry that you were in Vietnam. I know that was horrible. But it's absolutely irrelevant in terms of how you decide to spend the rest of your life.'" Once they see that they have a choice, they can learn not to dwell on thoughts that increase their depressed feelings. This psychotherapeutic model is known as Psychology of Mind, or the Health Realization model, and was developed in the 1970s by psychologists George S. Pransky, Ph.D., and Roger C. Mills, Ph.D., based on the ideas of theosophist Sydney Banks.

**Resources** For information about Psychology of Mind, see the website www.psychologyofmind.com; or contact Pransky and Associates, P.O. Box 506, LaConner, WA 98257; tel: 360-466-5200.

Dr. Weeks notes, though, that the cellular terrain and the psychological work operate in converse relationship to each other. "It's very hard to think your way out of depression without the biochemical support, and very hard to have the biochemical do anything unless you think your way out of it," he says.

When it comes to the spiritual realm, Dr. Weeks believes "that the spirit informs the soul, the soul informs the vitality (the life forces), and the life forces inform the physical body, more so than vice versa. I think we're fundamentally spiritual beings trying to make the world a better place, and basically learning how to love. To focus on the material is to miss the game."

He explains to his patients that spirit requires that they figure out what they want to do with their life. He asks them, "Why are you alive? How are you going to mean something with your life? Who are you going to help?" These are spiritual questions and not having answered them can be a component of mental illness, says Dr. Weeks. "Maybe a deficiency of doing something valuable in their own eyes, not in my judgmental eyes, but in *their* eyes, contributed to their illness."

Dr. Weeks is in agreement with Dr. Klinghardt (chapter 3) that healing happens faster from the spiritual level downward. "Whether it's homeopathy or talk therapy or something else, we can affect the physical body more from the top down than from the bottom up." This is not license to neglect treatment at the physical level, however. "To simply do the top down, and ignore the fact that the person's got a zinc deficiency, or an essential fatty acid deficiency, you're stepping on the gas and the brake," he says. His approach is to take care of the various factors concurrently.

## Bringing Light to the Darkness

One of the issues in depression is a light metabolism problem, according to Dr. Weeks. By this, he is not simply referring to seasonal affective disorder (SAD). Light metabolism refers to how the substance of light is handled in the body. He notes that oils (a category that includes fats and essential fatty acids) are an integral part of this subject. As discussed in chapter 2, deficiency in essential fatty acids can be a factor in mood disorders. While research has established this link, very few scientists or healing professionals are investigating the issue of light metabolism and the relationship between light and oils. Here is how Dr. Weeks explains the relationship and its significance for mental well-being:

> "On the physical level, what you have with every mental illness is a phospholipid spectrum disorder, as Dr. David Horrobin so elegantly describes in his textbook *Phospholipid Spectrum Disorder in Psychiatry* [Marius Press, 1999].
>
> "At the biochemical level, cell membrane abnormalities (phospholipid disturbance) are directly implicated in mental illness. But what does that mean in terms of light metabolism? What have oils to do with light? What have light and oil to do with mood disorders in general, and the black mood—melancholia—or depression in particular? These questions can be understood on the biochemical level as well as on the metaphysical level.
>
> "*Phos* is Greek for 'light,' and 'lipid' means 'oil,' so one could restate the word 'phospholipid' as 'lighted oil.' The ancients taught 'All life from light.' Yet today we smear on sunscreen immoderately and hide from the source of our life. Balance in light exposure is critically important.
>
> "We know that human blood levels of phosphorous decrease with diminished light exposure. Of course, other substances aside from oils have strong relationships to light: vitamin D (rickets), iron (flint sparks), and magnesium (chlorophyll metabolism). These substances comprise partial remedies for many mental illnesses including depression.
>
> "How do we see a role for light metabolism in mental illnesses? Consider that SAD, a relatively newly minted

mental illness, is light-dependent. Disruptions in light metabolism also contribute to sleep disruption, which itself directly contributes to mental illnesses, most notably mania and depression. So, we see that light metabolism plays a role in depression.

"What about the role of oil in mental illness? Oil has served thoughout our human development as a dependable source of light. Oil is the least terrestrial of our physical substances; its hydrogen is the 'lightest' of all elements and therefore has the least relationship to the earth. Oils have always been used to anoint kings, not for comfort alone but also to enhance the king's ability to receive cosmic wisdom from heaven for the benefit of his subjects on Earth. Sixty percent of the brain's dry weight is oil. Thus the term 'fat and happy.' Yet American consumers are taught to be terrified of oils in their diet. Patients tell me that these low-fat diets 'drive me crazy.' I do not discourage my patients from eating organic fatty foods as long as they are also getting regular exercise and minding their cardiovascular health.

"Metaphysically, one can think of depression as a biochemical imbalance of phospholipids that manifests as a static-riddled connection to the divine or spiritual world. Bliss and joy depend, in large part, upon protecting one's connection to the spiritual world, not only by creating spiritual meaning in one's life, but by eating 'enlightened' oils. The ubiquitous phospholipid membranes, literally our custom agents for all cell to cell communication, are built from a diet rich in essential fatty acids. Add to these health-giving organic oils a healthy dose of other light-filled nutrients (vitamin D, magnesium, vitamin C, iron) and you are creating a well-tuned instrument of reception to the spiritual world which is simply not conducive to depressed moods."

In cases of depression, Dr. Weeks often uses an anthroposophic remedy that operates primarily in this arena of light metabolism. It is a combination of meteoric iron, phosphorus, and quartz. "This is a remedy that gives courage and encouragement in the form of meteoric iron," he says. "Iron is that substance that, when you strike it, what happens? You get light. Hidden within this depressed, dark substance is light. We have a light-filled, dark stone." Phosphorus glows in the dark and also spontaneously catches fire when it is exposed to air. Quartz is transparent, "an inspirational substance that brings flexibility." The remedy facilitates the emergence of these qualities in the person taking it. It works on a psychospiritual level to shine light into the dark corners of depression.

 For information about anthroposophic medicine, contact the Anthroposophic Press; P.O. Box 960, Herndon, VA 20172-0960; tel: 703-661-1594 or 800-856-8664; website: www.anthropress.org. For referral to practitioners, contact the Physicians' Association for Anthroposophical Medicine (PAAM), 1923 Geddes Avenue, Ann Arbor, MI 48104-1797; tel: 734-930-9462; website: www.paam.net.

Another therapeutic modality that Dr. Weeks has found highly effective in bringing light into his depressive patients, even those with intractable depression, is apitherapy (*api* means 'bee'), which entails injections of bee venom. Apitherapy stimulates circulation, which is always beneficial in a disorder characterized by a sluggish system, as is the case with depression. In spiritual terms, bee venom comes from "a creature of light that flies in the light and is basically entirely organized by light forces," Dr. Weeks explains. "The venom is, I would say, the closest thing to substantial light. Not only are we delivering light forces, but we're delivering a bit of light with bee venom therapy."

## Joseph: Lifetime Depression

Joseph, 56, had not been happy since childhood. He first began seeing psychiatrists when he was in college and had been on every category of antidepressant, none of which were really helpful. Despite his depression, he became a high-functioning executive, but he never felt that his job, family, or even his life was meaningful or fun. Everything was duty. He was also plagued by insomnia. He occasionally had to take time off from work because of his condition, but for the most part he continued his career.

When Prozac hit the market, Joseph tried it and got some immediate benefit, but then became much worse, more agitated and more angry. His doctor switched him to another SSRI antidepressant. He had been suicidal for the past seven years, but at that point he became even more so. The recommendation was electroconvulsive therapy (ECT; formerly known as shock treatment). Joseph didn't want that.

It was then that he sought Dr. Weeks' help. Suicidal, separated from his family, in danger of losing his job, Joseph had by that time been on medication for depression for more than 30 years.

When Joseph came in for his first appointment, he was angry at everybody. Dr. Weeks talked about the mad-sad-bad situation, that "bad people are really mad people who are really sad people." In Joseph's case, the act of suicide was the bad, and being angry at everybody was the mad. So what was the sad? Joseph, who had been through a lot of psychiatry, started going over what his mother didn't do for him.

Dr. Weeks introduced the concept of Psychology of Mind. "I'm sorry that happened to you," he said to Joseph. "You're a human being and, by definition, you don't have to let that affect you. Why do you choose to let it affect you?" They talked from that perspective at first, and then at the next appointment began to deal with the physical level, restoring the milieu.

In addition to his depression and insomnia, Joseph had physical problems. He didn't exercise and ate fast-burning junk food, when he ate at all. He had heartburn, for which he was taking an antacid. He also suffered from chronic arthritis.

Blood tests revealed that he was very low in all of the amino acids, as well as other nutrients. Dr. Weeks started him on vitamin B injections and the appropriate vitamin and mineral supplements for his deficiencies. As the antacid he was taking would interfere with the absorption of any nutrients his poor diet could yield, Dr. Weeks gave him instead aloe vera, as a natural stomach aid, and licorice extract, which is helpful for acid reflux and heartburn. To address the chronic arthritis, Joseph began taking protease enzymes between meals; when taken on an empty stomach, these enzymes act on sites of inflammation, cleaning up cellular debris and helping to reduce the inflammation. At Dr. Weeks' request, he also drank a lot of water to help his body detoxify and began to exercise regularly.

Joseph's energy came back after about three days of the vitamin B shots and he reported that he felt better than he had in his whole life. "If there is anything that I would like to have up in neon lights, it is 'Ask your doctor about vitamin B shots,'" comments Dr. Weeks. "There's no excuse for this not being available."

To address Joseph's depression on a psychospiritual plane, Dr. Weeks gave him anthroposophic remedies: the classic meteoric iron, phosphorus, and quartz combination, discussed previously; and *Argentum* (silver). He also started him on bee venom, beginning with the homeopathic form, *Apis mellifera.* Later, Joseph got bee venom injections, which he found energizing. He liked the feeling that the injections gave him in his body. "Interestingly enough, he described it as a white light," says Dr. Weeks. That is in keeping with the role of both apitherapy and these specific anthroposophic remedies as antidepressant light therapy.

Within four months, Joseph was off his antidepressant as well as his arthritis medication. He continues to give himself the vitamin B shots twice a week. (Dr. Weeks teaches his patients how to administer the shots themselves so they are not dependent on him and can reduce the cost.) He also takes his individualized protocol of vitamins and minerals and gets regular exercise, which has become a hobby for him. All of this, along with having changed his eating habits and drinking plenty of water, has led to him feeling good in his body.

With the lifting of his depression, the circumstances of his life improved. He is now back at work and back with his family. Joseph found that the Psychology of Mind approach was helpful for him. At times when he starts feeling himself getting depressed, he acknowledges that the thoughts that are bringing him down are volitional and reminds himself that he can either dwell on them or not.

Joseph has chosen not to look much at the spiritual aspect of his depression, says Dr. Weeks. "He's just glad to be done with it." In Dr. Weeks' experience, however, unanswered spiritual questions have a way of surfacing again. Unfortunately, that may be in the form of serious illness, providing another opportunity for the person to explore the spiritual issues. "Rudolf Steiner said that human beings learn things in two ways," concludes Dr. Weeks. "Number one, we learn by our thinking. Number two, what we don't gather and understand through our thinking, we learn thanks to illness." Thus, depression and other illness can be seen to contain a gift, if we choose to accept it.

# 5 Energy Medicine I:
## Traditional Chinese Medicine

From the perspective of traditional Chinese medicine (TCM), depression, or any other disorder, results from a disturbance in energy flow in the body. That disturbance produces effects in the person's mind and spirit as well as on the physical level because body, mind, and spirit are inseparable, says Ira J. Golchehreh, L.Ac., O.M.D., whose practice is based in San Rafael, California. All three operate on energy and are fed by the same source, so all three are affected when the energy becomes imbalanced. By restoring proper energy flow in the body, TCM treatment thus helps restore balance in mind and spirit as well as body.

Many people in the West do not understand that traditional Chinese medicine, of which acupuncture is a component, is a complex system and requires as rigorous, if not more rigorous, training as Western medicine in order to be practiced correctly. The programs at the better traditional Chinese medical schools take eight years to complete. Dr. Golchehreh is a master of TCM, having trained with professors from the Shanghai Medical School, which is considered the Harvard Medical School of Chinese medicine. He has treated tens of thousands of patients in the twenty years that he has been practicing and can reverse many intractable conditions that other forms of medicine have been unable to treat.

While every individual is unique, there are certain kinds of energy imbalances that typically accompany depression, Dr.

Golchehreh says. Before we look at those patterns, let's get a better understanding of TCM and the energy it addresses.

## What Is Traditional Chinese Medicine?

Traditional Chinese medicine was developed more than five thousand years ago in China and is still the predominant medical system used in that country today. It is also now widely practiced in the United States and other Western countries. The primary treatment modalities of TCM are acupuncture and Chinese herbal medicine. TCM is a form of energy, or vibrational medicine, in that it is based on the flow of vital energy (*qi,* pronounced *chee*) in the body along energy channels known as meridians.

Another term for energy medicine is "molecular medicine," says Dr. Golchehreh. "When you look at the human being, you have to look at the molecular biology, the energy flow in the body, and the energy that is causing the vibrational weight between the cells and tissues."

Energy travels through the body along the meridians, which supply energy to organs, nerves, and other tissue. There are 12 primary meridians relating to the organs or organ systems, each bearing the name of the main organ it supplies, as in the Lung meridian, Heart meridian, Liver meridian, and Large Intestine meridian. In addition, there are two general meridians, the Governing Vessel and the Conception Vessel, as well as subsidiary energy channels.

**From the perspective of traditional Chinese medicine (TCM), depression, or any other disorder, results from a disturbance in energy flow in the body. That disturbance produces effects in the person's mind and spirit as well as on the physical level because body, mind, and spirit are inseparable, says Ira J. Golchehreh, L.Ac., O.M.D. By restoring proper energy flow in the body, TCM treatment thus helps restore balance in mind and spirit as well as body.**

Imbalances in energy flow can be excesses, deficiencies, or stagnation, and affect organs and systems throughout the body. TCM describes these imbalances and the attendant disharmony in the body in terms of natural world attributes such as heat, fire, cold, dampness, or dryness. These reflect the dominance of one or the other of the two essential qualities of qi: yin and yang. Yin is watery, dark, and calming, while yang is fiery, bright, and energizing. The names TCM uses to describe health conditions often have a poetic ring to them, as in Upflaming of Deficient Fire and Disorders of the Spirit Gate.

A doctor of Chinese medicine diagnoses the status of energy flow in a patient via the pulses, appearance of the tongue, and other physical and mien indications that practitioners are trained to observe. The pulses are not the Western medicine pulse as in heart rate, but distinct pulses corresponding to the organs and meridians. The energy qualities of the various pulses are described in language such as wiry, thready, choppy, rapid, slow, floating, tight, and slippery. The quality signals to the practitioner the energy status of the organ and meridian.

As treatment, acupuncture and Chinese herbs are administered to address the specific energy imbalances of the patient: to raise deficient energy, reduce excess energy, or remove blockages producing energy stagnation.

In acupuncture, thin needles are shallowly inserted into the skin at strategic points (acupoints) along the meridian(s) requiring treatment, and left in place for an average of a half-hour. This is a painless procedure, and patients often fall asleep while the needles are doing their work.

Acupuncture has application to a broad range of conditions, but has become particularly known in the United States for its efficacy in relieving pain.

 **In the United States, there are thousands of acupuncturists and doctors of traditional Chinese medicine. These medical practices require extensive training. Ask practitioners for information about their training and avoid those who have only taken**

a quick course. One organization that can help you locate an acupuncturist in your area is the National Certification Commission for Acupuncture and Oriental Medicine (NCCAOM), 11 Canal Center Plaza, Suite 300, Alexandria, VA 22314; tel: 703-548-9004; website: www.nccaom.org.

## Types of Depression in TCM

Chinese medicine classifies depression as one of two different kinds, according to symptoms and what is occurring in the energy meridians and the organs, as determined by TCM diagnosis, says Dr. Golchehreh. One is called Deficient Type; this is depression, ranging from mild to severe. The other kind is called Excess Type; this is what is known in Western medicine as bipolar disorder, characterized by the classic ups and downs in mood. In this book, we look only at Deficient Type depression. (For coverage of Excess Type, see the author's *The Natural Medicine Guide to Bipolar Disorder,* [Hampton Roads, 2003].)

Dr. Golchehreh cites three subcategories of the Deficient Type depression: (1) Disturbed Mind; (2) Deficiency of Heart and Spleen; and (3) Upflaming of Deficient Fire.

In addition to the specific treatments cited for each type, Dr. Golchehreh also gives all of his depressed patients hypericin (the active constituent in St. John's wort) and two homeopathic remedies (a homeopathic serotonin-dopamine combination, and Antidepression Drops, a formula containing homeopathic lithium, serotonin, a pineal preparation, *Aurum metallicum,* and *Natrum muriaticum*). "It is important to make sure that the person is getting as much benefit as possible as quickly as possible," says Dr. Golchehreh, particularly if there is any risk of suicide.

### Disturbed Mind

The name of this category reflects the presenting symptoms, but the root of the disturbance is deficient energy on the Heart meridian. This type of depression is characterized by restlessness, moodiness, and an inability to concentrate. The person feels sad,

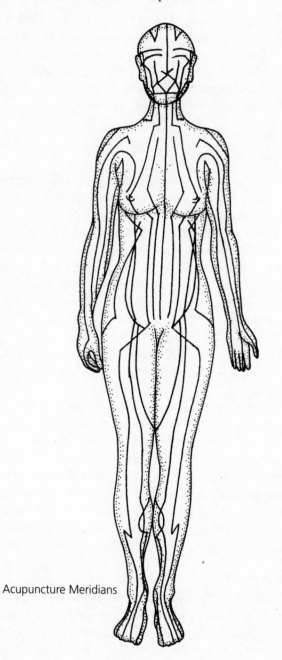

Acupuncture Meridians

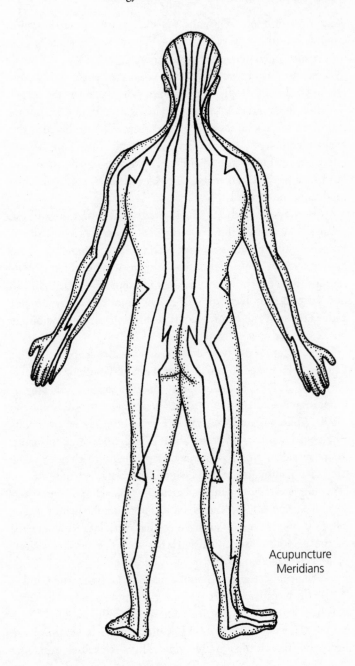

Acupuncture
Meridians

has a constant desire to cry, and sighs frequently. Insomnia is also a problem in this type of depression. The tongue is white with a thin coating. The pulses are weak and wiry.

The mind and heart are closely connected energetically, says Dr. Golchehreh. "People who have heart disease, for example, get forgetful; the mind cannot concentrate. You get symptoms of forgetfulness with malfunction of the heart. This is because the Heart meridian controls the nervous system, which controls the mind." In the case of the Disturbed Mind type of depression, you must look to the Heart meridian to correct the energy deficiency producing the problem.

An energy imbalance in the Heart meridian can throw off the balance of neurotransmitters in the brain, notes Dr. Golchehreh. Proper chemistry can be restored by restoring the function of the Heart meridian. This relationship explains why psychiatric medications that attempt to correct the biochemistry of the brain do not solve the problem of depression: antidepressants do not address the root energy problem that threw the neurotransmitters out of balance in the first place.

Treatment for this type of depression involves acupuncture and Chinese herbs aimed at "tonifying the heart and soothing the unstable mind," as Dr. Golchehreh puts it. This means strengthening or supporting the function of the heart and stabilizing or calming the mind. While acupuncture treatment focuses on the Heart meridian, it will likely treat other meridians as well, because an imbalance in one meridian produces energy flow problems in others.

Acupuncture treatment of a meridian has far-reaching effects. "It is important to remember," says Dr. Golchehreh, "that when we're treating the Heart meridian, it is not only the meridian, but all of the nerves that are supplied by that meridian. It's a network of the nervous system, which carries the biochemistry that is behind the function of that organ."

The goal of strengthening the heart and calming the mind is "to get the heart back in charge, controlling the mind." The herbs that help with this are a licorice and jujube combination. "These are the herbs traditionally used in Chinese medicine to tonify the heart and smooth the unstable mind," Dr. Golchehreh explains.

# TCM Types of Depression

## Disturbed Mind

Symptoms: restlessness, moodiness, inability to concentrate, insomnia, desire to cry, frequent sighing

Pulses: weak, wiry

Tongue: white with a thin coating

Primary meridian(s) involved: heart

Treatment: tonify the heart, smooth the unstable mind

Herbs: licorice, jujube

Other remedies: hypericin and homeopathic medicine

## Deficiency of Heart and Spleen

Symptoms: "deep pensiveness," excessive thinking and worrying, emotional fearfulness, heart palpitations, sleep problems, pale face, fatigue, low energy, reduced or no appetite

Pulses: very thin and weak

Tongue: pale but not white, with a very thin coating

Primary meridian(s) involved: heart and spleen

Treatment: tonify the heart and spleen

Herbs: ginseng, longan

Other remedies: hypericin and homeopathic medicine

## Upflaming of Deficient Fire

Symptoms: dizziness, heart palpitations, sleep problems, high restlessness, quickness to anger, weak and sore lower back, irregular menstruation

Pulse: wiry, fiery, deficient, and thin

Tongue: red

Primary meridian(s) involved: kidney

Treatment: tonify the yin, clear the heat, tranquilize the mind

Herbs: lycium, chrysanthemum, rehmannia

Other remedies: hypericin and homeopathic medicine

## Deficiency of Heart and Spleen

The second minor depression type is deficiency of the function of the heart and the spleen, deficiency on the Heart and Spleen meridians. The presenting symptoms in this case are "deep pensiveness," excessive thinking, and worrying. "This type of person is always emotionally fearful," says Dr. Golchehreh. "Because of that, and because he's thinking too much and worrying too much, he gets heart palpitations." All of this causes sleep problems.

The constant worrying (and the compromised heart function) is reflected in a paleness of the face. "Since the heart is not pumping the blood correctly, and the spleen is not providing the heart with the blood that it needs, it causes fatigue, low energy," says Dr. Golchehreh. The deficiency of the spleen also results in reduced or no appetite. The tongue is pale but not white, with a very thin coating. The pulses are very thin and weak.

Treatment focuses on tonifying or strengthening the heart and the spleen. "Since the spleen provides the blood and the heart provides the qi, strengthening the heart and the spleen makes the qi and the blood strong," explains Dr. Golchehreh. Acupuncture treats the Heart and Spleen meridians to correct the deficient energy flow. The herbs used are those known to strengthen the heart, spleen, and qi. A ginseng and longan combination is a good one for this, according to Dr. Golchehreh. He also uses a ginseng nutritive combination, which contains all the different kinds of ginseng.

## Upflaming of Deficient Fire

The third deficient syndrome type is the Upflaming of Deficient Fire. The primary symptoms with this kind are dizziness because of the deficiency. The deficient fire aspect results in heart palpitations, sleep problems, high restlessness, and quickness to anger. In addition, the lumbar region of the back becomes weak and sore; in the female, menstruation becomes very irregular. The tongue is red. The pulses are wiry and fiery, but at the same time, deficient and thin.

*Upflaming* and *deficient* seem to be contradictory, but Dr.

Golchehreh explains the condition in this way: "If the energy is deficient, it should not be coming up. But when there is fire, it means the yin is depleted." (Remember that all energy has complementary yin and yang aspects.) "With the yin depleted, the yang is in excess. The yang, or fire, is allowed to come to the surface. The yin is more like providing the water to the system. When we have a deficient yin, there's no cooling effect and it causes the fire to upflame." Thus, Upflaming of Deficient Fire (excess fire born of deficient yin).

To treat this condition, it is necessary to tonify the yin, to bring up the water to cool down the fire, so to speak. In this type of depression, the Kidney meridian is the site of the deficient yin—in TCM, the kidneys are considered to hold the essence of life—so it is the focus of acupuncture treatment. Acupuncture and herbs work together to tonify the yin, clear the heat, and tranquilize the mind. Indicated herbs for this are lycium, chrysanthemum, and rehmannia.

## Causes of Energy Disturbance

The flow of vital energy (qi) in the body can be thrown out of balance—become excessive, deficient, blocked, or stagnant—by influences on the physical, psychological, or spiritual levels. Biochemical, functional, or metabolic factors can be involved. A poor diet, organ malfunction, toxicity, and stress all affect energy flow in the body. It is the chicken or the egg issue, however. Did a psychological trauma disrupt the flow of qi, which in turn threw off the body's biochemistry, for example, or did a poor diet result in biochemical deficiencies, which led to energy disturbance and psychological problems?

While stress can produce many symptoms, it is particularly an issue with the deficient type of depression, says Dr. Golchehreh. For someone with that underlying energy state, stress can easily trigger depression. Genetics may be a factor as well. You can inherit a tendency for your qi to be deficient (or in excess), he notes. "That genetic tendency could go back centuries." This inheritance can set you up for depression.

The factors that affect qi can be internal or external. Just as the body, mind, and spirit are related within a human being, human beings are also elements in the environment, says Dr. Golchehreh. "You're definitely under the influence of what's going on outside, physically, chemically, and in every other way. Your body chemistry has a tendency to fluctuate accordingly. We are not individual parts. We are a part of the whole. That's why the pollution in the air, for example, could also cause some kind of problems internally, like in the lung, the heart, and the liver."

In acupuncture, as with other natural medicine modalities, there are layers of healing. Underneath the energy imbalances that are producing the presenting symptoms may be other energy imbalances that can be addressed once the "top" layer is removed, explains Dr. Golchehreh. What is presenting on top is the acute aspect, and what is underlying is the chronic. "So there are different layers of a problem that affect a person psychologically, mentally, and physically," he concludes.

The complexity of influences involved in "mental" disorders such as depression make it imperative to consider the person as a whole—body, mind, and spirit—in treatment, as TCM does. "You cannot just give them a drug and send them home," says Dr. Golchehreh.

## Rosa: Twelve Weeks Reversed Twelve Years

Rosa, 50, had been suffering from moderate depression for 12 years when she consulted Dr. Golchehreh, not for her depression initially but for uterine fibroids. During the intake, she told him about her depression and that she had tried antidepressants but was not happy with the results.

Her depression, which rated a six or seven on a scale of ten, with ten being the most severe, was interfering with her life. "This kind of depression (the Deficiency of Heart and Spleen type) causes the person to lose their memory, in most cases, which impacts on their job duties," he notes. This was the case with Rosa, who was a writer and educator. The depression had caused her to pull away from people and, when she wasn't at work, she spent most of her time alone. She was frequently tearful and prone to emotional outbursts.

Rosa demonstrated "organic disharmony, too," Dr. Golchehreh recalls, as evidenced by heart palpitations that woke her up at night, insomnia, and the fibroids, which were causing gastrointestinal distress and a sensation of pressure in the abdomen and chest. Due to the insomnia, she was constantly tired.

Her depression was worse in the winter. She felt the loneliness of her isolated life more at that time of year, too. Diminished light obviously contributed to her depression, but TCM looks at the issue in a different way from the Western medical analysis of seasonal affective disorder (SAD). In Chinese medicine, light has to do with the heart, explains Dr. Golchehreh. In Rosa's case, the lack of light aggravated her Heart meridian deficiency, which in turn deepened her depression.

As is standard in cases of Defiency of Heart and Spleen, Rosa's pulses were very weak and thin, or thready. This reflected the fact that she was so "deficient and introverted, pulled into herself," Dr. Golchehreh observes. Her Liver meridian also needed treatment. As noted earlier, imbalance in one meridian often produces disturbance in the energy flow in one or more of the others because of the interrelated nature of the meridian system. Problems on the Liver meridian can cause both depression and uterine fibroids.

Rosa received acupuncture treatments once a week, along with a Chinese herbal formula of ginseng and longan, which is a classic combination for this type of deficient depression. After a month of treatment, Dr. Golchehreh gave her another herbal formula, this one containing all the ginsengs, to "make her stronger internally, and help with the organ deficiency." Rosa also took the hypericin and homeopathic remedies that Dr. Golchehreh gives in all cases of depression. The acupuncture and herbs worked together to tonify the Heart, Spleen, and Liver meridians and restore the energy balance in her body.

The first few sessions didn't produce much of a difference, which was to be expected, according to Dr. Golchehreh. After the readjustment effected through acupuncture, "it takes a little bit of time for the organs to go back to normal functioning," he says. This is especially true in a case of chronic depression like Rosa's.

After three or four visits, things shifted for Rosa. The heart palpitations disappeared and she was able to sleep. With better sleep, she wasn't as tired in the morning. Her depression lifted greatly, dropping to around a three on a scale of one to ten. She began to engage more with the world around her. Her gastrointestinal complaints had improved as well.

"The heart and spleen are very important in terms of the functioning of the other organs in the body," notes Dr. Golchehreh. When these are very deficient, as they were in Rosa's case, all of the other organs will be disharmonized as well. As Rosa had had this problem for more than a decade, it could be expected that restoring harmony to the body would take a while. Dr. Golchehreh tells patients with a chronic problem like hers that it will likely be six weeks before they see a significant change (six weeks for major changes in a chronic health condition is impressive as it is).

Rosa, however, made excellent progress in just a few weeks. Dr. Golchehreh credits this to her compliance (she religiously took her herbs and kept her acupuncture appointments) and to the psychotherapy she started at the same time, which served as an excellent complement to the energy rebalancing of TCM. Rosa stopped seeing the psychiatrist who gave her antidepressant medications and switched to a psychotherapist who helped her look at some of the emotional and pscyhological issues in her depression. Given the relationship of body, mind, and spirit, it was important for Rosa to look at all the possible contributing factors to her energy imbalance and long-term depression.

After 12 acupuncture sessions, Rosa was doing fine, with no signs of any of her original symptoms. (Dr. Golchehreh notes that the uterine fibroids may have still been there, but were no longer producing any symptoms.) The depression of many years was almost down to zero. She felt she just needed to continue with psychotherapy to address the residuals. The heart palpitations and insomnia had not returned, and her pulses indicated that the energy on her Heart and Spleen meridians was no longer deficient, and all her other organs were restored to harmonious function again.

# 6 Energy Medicine II: Homeopathy

In addition to acupuncture, another form of energy medicine is particularly effective in the treatment of depression: homeopathy. Homeopathy is similar to flower essence therapy (see next chapter) in that the medicines they employ do not contain biochemical components of the plants (or other substances, in the case of homeopathy) from which they are derived, but rather encapsulate their energetic qualities. The medicines help restore the individual's energy (or vital force) to its natural equilibrium and thus return balance to the body, mind, and spirit.

Judyth Reichenberg-Ullman, N.D., L.C.S.W., of Edmonds, Washington, is an internationally known naturopathic and homeopathic physician. She and her husband, Robert Ullman, N.D., teach, lecture, and have written numerous books together, including *Prozac Free: Homeopathic Alternatives to Conventional Drug Therapies*. Their column on homeopathic treatment has run in the esteemed journal *Townsend Letter for Doctors and Patients* since 1990.

Dr. Reichenberg-Ullman went into homeopathy because of her interest in mental health. In her early career as a psychiatric social worker, she worked on a locked psychiatric ward, in emergency rooms, nursing homes, halfway houses, and people's homes. "I saw the whole spectrum, and the suffering was terrible," she recalls. "I didn't see conventional medicine as having a magic bullet for most of these people. With the degree of side effects they were experiencing [from medications], I thought there must be something better."[107]

Dr. Reichenberg-Ullman discovered that "something better" in homeopathy, as did her husband. They wrote *Prozac Free* to share their discovery of an effective alternative to medications for depression and other psychiatric disorders. "As shown by the many patients we have treated successfully, we believe we have found a method that can transform the lives of many people," she states.[108]

"Certainly homeopathy can't help everybody, but the number of people that can be helped with these impairing mental and emotional conditions is incredibly gratifying."

For depression, homeopathy is not only "safe, long-lasting, and highly effective," she says, but it also "has the potential to alleviate your physical problems as well as your depression."[109] This is because homeopathy addresses the underlying imbalance that is responsible for all of a person's symptoms. The imbalance occurs on an energetic level, which is why an energy medicine such as homeopathy is so effective in restoring balance. Let's look more closely at the concept of energy imbalance.

We are energetic organisms, or energy-modulated organisms, explains Dr. Reichenberg-Ullman, and that energy is our vital force. "The vital force of each person, because of their makeup, has a certain susceptibility. Due to that susceptibility there are going to be certain factors that trigger an imbalance or symptoms in that person." The individual susceptibility is why genetics are not inevitably predetermining. For example, in a family in which one parent has bipolar disorder, which research has shown to have a genetic component, one of the children develops the illness and the others don't. That one child was susceptible in some way. The same is true of nonpsychiatric illnesses, Dr. Reichenberg-Ullman points out, citing epidemics as an example. Even in virulent epidemics, there are people who are not susceptible and do not contract the illness, she notes.

In the case of depression, certain triggers or causes can produce it, but the person has to have a susceptibility, or vulnerability, in those areas. Such triggers or causes include, according to Dr. Reichenberg-Ullman, genetics, lack of nurturing or other environmental factors in childhood, challenging life events, hormonal issues, side effects of prescription medication, and imbalance in neurotransmitters.[110] These factors will likely not produce depression, however, unless the person's vital force is compromised. Some of the factors, such as hormonal or neurotransmitter problems, are directly caused by an underlying vital force imbalance. With others, there is a cyclical relationship; lack of nurturing in childhood and challenging life events, for example, disturb the vital force, which in turn sets one up for depression, which in turn further weakens the vital force.

*In the case of depression, certain triggers or causes can produce it, but the person has to have a susceptibility, or vulnerability, in those areas. Such triggers or causes include, according to Dr. Reichenberg-Ullman, genetics, lack of nurturing or other environmental factors in childhood, challenging life events, hormonal issues, side effects of prescription medication, and imbalance in neurotransmitters.*

"It's important to realize that the vital force or the energetic equilibrium of that individual is the bottom line," says Dr. Reichenberg-Ullman. "When there is an imbalance, a disturbance underneath the surface of the lake, then there are ripples that go out. Those ripples can manifest in any number of ways. One of those ripples could end up being a biochemical imbalance, an imbalance in neurotransmitters."

Scientific consensus currently holds that neurotransmitter problems are the factor behind depression and other mental disorders. In actuality, the research supporting this is "still more theoretical than they would make it out to be," says Dr. Reichenberg-Ullman. In her view, a deeper imbalance in a person's energetic equilibrium is what throws neurotransmitter supply and function out of balance.

Thus, simply attempting to correct the neurotransmitter problem is not getting to the real source of the mental disorder. "You have to deal with that underlying disturbance, or else it's like putting your finger in the dike, which I think is what, to a large degree, conventional medicine is doing." She cites the use of Prozac as an example of putting the finger in the dike.

The implication of vital force in depression is clear when you consider that "probably the most important factor triggering depression is a lack of passion or purpose," says Dr. Reichenberg-Ullman. You could also call this a lack of meaning or direction. "If more people had deeply satisfying work, relationships, spiritual lives, and a genuine sense of purpose, we could guarantee that the incidence of depression and need for Prozac would be much diminished," she states.[111]

Tragic or traumatic life events can interfere with your sense of purpose. Grief over the death of a spouse, for example, zaps your vital force, which, if not restored, can produce a lack of purpose, which is in turn a trigger for chronic depression. Homeopathy can provide support at these times and serve as an intervention that keeps the cycle from escalating. Dr. Reichenberg-Ullman recalls her days of ministering to people whose family members died in the emergency room. "The psychiatric social workers are wonderful, but all they have to offer is antianxiety medications like Xanax," she notes. "If there were somebody there offering homeopathy as one of the alternatives, it would be tremendous."

Homeopathy can restore balance thrown off by what Dr. Reichenberg-Ullman calls the tumults or turmoils of life. Psychotherapy, while providing important tools and support, does not necessarily address the vital force disequilibrium caused by these tumults. People who have been through a challenging event or are in a difficult life situation may, despite therapy, still have a lot of fear and not feel in control of their lives. "Homeopathy can bring them into balance in a way that they didn't think was possible," she states.

Like many natural medicine physicians, Dr. Reichenberg-Ullman regards symptoms, whether mental, emotional, or physical,

## The Benefits of Homeopathic Treatment

Dr. Reichenberg-Ullman cites the following benefits of constitutional homeopathic treatment.[112] Homeopathy:

- treats the whole person

- treats the root of the problem

- treats each person as an individual

- uses natural, nontoxic medicines

- is considered safe and does not have the side effects of prescription drugs

- heals physical, mental, and emotional symptoms

- uses medicines, one dose of which works for months or years rather than hours

- uses inexpensive medicines

- is cost effective.

as an individual's attempt to cope with the underlying disturbance. The body has its own wisdom, and symptoms are the ways in which a particular person adapts to the imbalance in her vital force. The beauty of homeopathy is that it goes to the heart of the matter and corrects the disturbance in the vital force. From that, all the other imbalances, including neurotransmitter and hormonal problems, correct as well. This is why homeopathy can address both your depression and whatever physical problems you are manifesting.

## What Is Homeopathy?

To understand *homeopathy*, it is helpful to consider the derivation of the word as well as that of *allopathy*, both of which were coined by the father of homeopathy, Dr. Samuel Hahnemann, in the late 1700s. A German physician and chemist who became increasingly frustrated with conventional medical practice, Dr. Hahnemann devoted himself to developing a safer, more effective approach to medicine. The result was homeopathy, which arose out of his discovery that illness can be treated by giving the patient a dilution of a plant that produces symptoms resembling those of the illness when given to a healthy person.

This principle, "let likes be cured with likes," became known as the Law of Similars. Dr. Hahnemann named this system of healing "homeopathy," a combination of the Greek *homoios* (similar) and *pathos* (suffering). At the same time, he dubbed conventional medicine *allopathy*, which means "opposite suffering," to reflect that model's approach of treating illness by giving an antidote to the symptoms, a medicine that produces the opposite effect from what the patient is suffering. (A laxative for constipation is an illustration of the allopathic approach; it produces diarrhea.)[113]

Homeopathic remedies can be employed as a simple remedy to address a certain transitory ailment or as a constitutional remedy to address the whole cluster of physical, psychological, and emotional characteristics—the constitution—of an individual patient. A constitutional remedy works to restore balance, and thus health, on all levels.

Homeopathic remedies are prepared through a process of dilution of plant, mineral, or animal substances, which results in a "potentized" remedy, one that contains the energy imprint of the substance rather than its biochemical components. This is why homeopathy falls into the category of energy medicine; it works on an energetic level to effect change in all aspects of a person and restore balance to the whole.

Paradoxically, the higher the number of dilutions, the greater the potency and the effects of the remedy. Thus the higher the potency number, the more powerful the remedy. Remedies used to treat a transitory condition are usually 6C, 12C, or 30C, relatively low-potency remedies. A constitutional remedy is often a 1M potency, which means it has been diluted a thousand times.

## Constitutional Treatment of Depression

Classical or constitutional homeopathic treatment is distinct from the use of homeopathic remedies for acute symptoms in that it employs a single remedy that addresses the particular and unique mental, emotional, and physical state of an individual. Dr. Reichenberg-Ullman explains it this way: "Each child, or adult, is much like a jigsaw puzzle. Once all of the pieces are assembled in their proper places, an image emerges that is distinct from other puzzles. It is the task of a homeopath to recognize that image and to match it to the corresponding image of one specific homeopathic medicine."[114]

The homeopath makes that match by considering the person's behaviors, feelings, attitudes, beliefs, likes, dislikes, physical symptoms, prenatal and birth history, family medical history, eating and sleeping patterns, and even dreams and fears.[115] By giving the remedy whose qualities match this unique cluster most closely, the homeopathic principle of "like cures like" is put into operation, and the remedy works to restore the person to balance. People may have one constitutional remedy that is their match throughout their life, or it may change over time, and a different constitutional remedy might then be required.

Homeopathy does not prescribe according to diagnostic labels, but rather according to the complete picture of the individual. Thus, there is no universal remedy for depression, and two people suffering from this disorder will likely require two entirely different remedies.

It's interesting to note that the qualities of the remedy that is the correct one for a person reflect their areas of susceptibility or vulnerability. "When a certain homeopathic medicine benefits a person, that tells me something about that person," observes Dr. Reichenberg-Ullman. "From understanding that homeopathic medicine, I know what kinds of conditions, whether mental, emotional, or physical, the person is likely to be susceptible to and what kinds they aren't. It often gives you a predictive capacity. Conventional medicine doesn't understand people deeply enough in most cases to be able to do that."

A single dose of a constitutional remedy is sometimes all that is needed at first. When the remedy is the correct one for an individual, changes can begin relatively quickly, within two to five weeks after taking the dose. (Some people experience changes in the first day, or even within hours.) If there are no changes within five weeks, that generally indicates that it is not the proper remedy. A remedy continues to work over time, anywhere from four months to a year or longer. Repeat doses may be necessary if there is a relapse of symptoms, or sometimes a different remedy may be called for.

Due to the way homeopathic remedies work, it is important to continue treatment for one to two years at least, states Dr. Reichenberg-Ullman. This does not necessarily entail frequent appointments with your homeopath, however. As stated, a single dose of a remedy works for some time.

While certain substances (notably coffee, menthol, camphor, and eucalyptus) can antidote homeopathic remedies in some sensitive individuals, prescription medications may not interfere with their function, and vice versa. (Topical steroids, antibiotics, and antifungals and oral antibiotics and cortisone products can be suppressive and are best used in consultation with your homeopath.[116]) Thus, you can pursue homeopathic treatment while continuing your medications or working with your prescribing doctor to phase them out when possible.

As a final note regarding the efficacy of homeopathy in treating depression, Dr. Reichenberg-Ullman states, "Homeopathic effectiveness is most limited by the skill, knowledge, and experience of the homeopath and the cooperation of the patient. The theory works, but it must be applied well and for a long enough time with sufficient expertise to produce results."[117]

 There are more than one thousand homeopaths in the United States, a small percentage of whom specialize in mental health. One source to help you find a qualified homeopath in your area is the Homeopathic Academy of Naturopathic Physicians (HANP), 12132 SE Foster Place, Portland, OR 97266; tel: 503-761-3298; website: www.healthy.net/hanp.

## Audrey: Lifting the Weight of the World

This case from the patient files of Dr. Reichenberg-Ullman illustrates how homeopathy can significantly help individuals suffering from depression.*

When Audrey, 59, consulted Dr. Reichenberg-Ullman, she was on Desipramine for depression. The drug was alleviating her mood trough, but if she tried to stop taking it, she plummeted into despair again. She was looking for another way to deal with the depression and anxiety that had plagued her intermittently in her adult life.

Depression ran in her family, and Audrey reports that her first severe episode occurred in her mid-twenties when both of her parents died in the space of six months, her father from an aneurysm and her mother from "a broken heart." The oldest of six children, Audrey felt responsible for her siblings but powerless to fix the situation for them. "I was filled with feelings of inadequacy," she says.

She married an alcoholic, but managed to keep herself and her life together until she divorced her husband at the age of 49. She plunged into another depression then. "I finally fell apart," she recalls, and realized "how inadequate I was to be in this world." Her job performance declined and she describes what she felt as despair, feeling lost, and not knowing what to do. Audrey had another, similar episode five years later when her finances "ran amok."

The third major episode, which brought her to Dr. Reichenberg-Ullman, was all too familiar. "My enthusiasm and zest for life have evaporated. I can't seem to hold things together," said Audrey. "My family is a mess. My son was recently hospitalized for depression. My daughter and I aren't communicating well. My sister is dying from ovarian cancer. I have a constant churning in my stomach from anxiety."

---

* This case study adapted, by permission of Judyth Reichenberg-Ullman, N.D., L.C.S.W., from her book, written with Robert Ullman, N.D., *Prozac Free: Homeopathic Alternatives to Conventional Drug Therapies* (Berkeley, CA: North Atlantic Books, 2002), pages 122–125.

Audrey was tired of being responsible, felt that her ambition was gone, and felt that she had failed in life. "I don't feel I've done a great job raising my family, and I've never been as successful in sales as I would have liked. I felt guilty about not spending enough time with the kids because of my work and for neglecting my work for the kids." Among her failures, she cited a fabric store business she started that went bankrupt, her failed marriage, and struggles with her weight. She was overweight and self-conscious about it for years.

"There's nothing I've ever excelled at doing," she said, adding, "not from lack of conscientiousness. I reproach myself for doing the wrong thing. There's a continual pressure on me to perform." As a child, Audrey had difficulty in school because she transposed letters. As an adult, it was hard for her to remember numbers, memorize information, and retain what she read.

Other facts about Audrey are that, as a young adult, she had acne, for which she took a lot of antibiotics, and she has had a lot of dental work, including two root canals and many gold fillings. As Audrey puts it, she has "a mouth full of gold."

Interestingly, Audrey's constitutional remedy was *Aurum metallicum* (gold), which is, as Dr. Reichenberg-Ullman explains, "a good medicine for depressed individuals who carry the burdens of others on their shoulders, have very high standards of performance, and rarely feel up to the task at hand." She adds, "It may or may not be a coincidence that Audrey's mouth was filled with gold."

In two months, Audrey was feeling great. "I don't cry anymore. I'm happy and don't feel overwhelmed. In fact I feel at peace. My life is much more in control." She even felt good during the holidays, a notoriously difficult time for depressed people. Audrey reported that the improvement had not been sudden, but had occurred gradually. The change was significant enough that her psychiatrist had lowered her Desipramine dosage, and Audrey planned to work with her to get off the drug completely.

Four months later, Audrey was still doing well and had decided to retire because work wasn't fun. She was enjoying spending time with her grandchildren and was in a "very compatible relationship," with plans for marriage.

Audrey needed two more doses of *Aurum,* once after some dental work and then again after she ate coffee ice cream and noticed she started feeling bad again. Dental work and coffee are known to antidote homeopathic medicine. People often overlook less obvious sources of coffee, as in coffee-flavored ice cream, yogurt, or candy.

A year after beginning homeopathic treatment, Audrey was still doing fine, her former problems with depression and anxiety gone.

# 7 Energy Medicine III: Flower Essence Therapy

Like homeopathy, flower essence therapy works on an energetic level to restore the equilibrium of the body, mind, and spirit. It does so by working with the issues that an individual human soul is facing, says Patricia Kaminski, co-director of the Flower Essence Society in Nevada City, California, and a renowned innovator in the field of flower essence therapy for more than 20 years (see "What Is Flower Essence Therapy?"). Viewed from this perspective, illness of any kind, including depression, offers an opportunity for the soul to grow.

"The approach of flower essence therapy is to recognize the dignity of the human soul and to recognize the capacity of the human soul to change and become stronger," she elaborates. "The soul isn't connected to the aging of the body, so even if you're 70 years old, you can still be developing from the point of view of the soul. What we want to look at when somebody is facing a crisis, when they present with depression, with anxiety, with an addiction, is what is it that the soul is really facing? . . . There's enormous capacity in the human spirit and the human soul to acquire skills for transforming what is a problem into a gift, if the therapy goes deep enough."

From this viewpoint, the biochemical imbalances found in depression are caused by the soul's distress. This is similar to Dr. Reichenberg-Ullman's explanation in the previous chapter of an imbalance in the vital force throwing off the biochemistry of the body. Just as addressing only the biochemistry will not cure depression because it does not deal with the problem of the energy imbalance, the flower essence model holds that a biochemical approach will not cure depression because it does not deal with the crisis in the soul.

The common interpretation of test results that reveal skewed brain chemistry is that if the doctor can manipulate the brain chemistry with medications, that will cure the illness. "While it is true that we can get some surface change by manipulating brain chemistry, we do not gain an insight into what is happening to the human soul," observes Kaminski. "The problem with the biochemical approach is that we haven't addressed why the person's brain dysfunction is there in the first place. From the point of view of flower essences, we're saying the soul is larger than the body. The brain is a receptor and a reflector for what is happening with our souls."

Kaminski notes that the cultural model is quite different when it comes to physical development of an individual versus psychological/soul development. She explains:

"We encourage those injured in sports to transform physical pain or stress, recognizing that a certain amount of challenge to the physical body is actually an opportunity to become stronger and more resilient. Even those severely injured in auto accidents or elderly patients with degenerative physical illnesses are assigned to rehabilitative programs premised on the idea that one's current condition of weakness or bodily pain can be overcome through physical therapy, strength training, and the like. By contrast, the current psychopharmaceutical model for the emotional health of the individual is quite truncated. We intervene earlier and earlier when someone is in emotional pain and distress, and we use biochemical therapies to 'fix' the problem at its current level of symptom manifestation, rather than encouraging further psychological development."

## What Is Flower Essence Therapy?

The use of flower essences is often dismissed in the United States, even by some alternative medicine practitioners, as a "lightweight" therapy that may be pleasing, but that has little therapeutic value. In actuality, flower essence therapy has the capability to stimulate profound change on a deep level. One reason for the misconception may be the general lack of understanding in this country about energy medicine.

To clarify another common misunderstanding, essential oils (aromatherapy) and flower essences are two very different kinds of medicine. While essential oils contain the biochemical components of the plants from which they are extracted, flower essences are closer to homeopathic remedies in nature, in that they are energetic imprints of their source. Another way of saying this is that a flower essence contains the life force of the flower.

A flower essence is made by sun-infusing the blossoms of a particular plant, bush, or tree in water. (This is a simplistic summary of the process, which involves timing the picking of the flowers according to life-cycle, environmental, and other factors.) The liquid is then diluted and potentized in a method similar to the preparation of homeopathic remedies, and preserved with brandy (or a nonalcoholic substance, if need be). The result is a highly diluted, potentized substance that embodies the energetic patterns of the flower from which it is made. This means that the therapeutic effects of flower essences are vibrational, or energetic.[118]

Despite Einstein and solid science demonstrating that matter is energy, the fact that you can contain energy in a liquid and influence human energy fields to help resolve ailments is not widely known. Yet, that is precisely what flower essence liquids do. When you take flower essences, the energy they contain affects your energy fields, which in turn has an impact on your physical, mental, emotional, and spiritual condition, as these aspects are all energy based.

The particular specialty of flower essences is the realm of emotions and attitudes, which have come to be accepted as exerting a powerful influence on health and ill health. As Edward Bach, the father of flower essence therapy, stated it, "Behind all disease lies our fears, our anxieties, our greed, our likes and dislikes."[119] By promoting energetic shifts in the mind and emotions, flower essences promote a return to health. Put simply, flower essences are "catalysts to mind-body wellness." Or you could say they act as a bridge between the realms of the physical and the spiritual, the body and the soul.[120]

In the 1930s, Dr. Bach, an English physician and homeopath, developed 38 different flower essences to address 38 different emotional-soul or psychological types. As an example of the "profile" associated with a remedy, the flower essence Willow is indicated for someone who, when out of balance, feels resentful, bitter, and envious of others, and adopts a "poor me" victim stance. Dr. Bach's remedies are still available today—the Bach Flower Remedies seen in health food stores everywhere.

The Flower Essence Society (FES) in Nevada City, California, headed by Kaminski and her husband, Richard Katz, has expanded on the work of Dr. Bach and significantly furthered the field of flower essences. Founded in 1979 by Katz, FES is a pioneer in flower essence research. In addition, Kaminski and Katz expanded on Bach's remedies, developing a line of more than 100 flower essences derived from North American plants. They developed the line (the FES brand) to expand the emotional repertoire of flower essences; to provide North Americans with essences derived from indigenous plants, which might better resonate with their healing issues; and to address the more complicated emotional and psychological makeup of people today.

There are many flower essence practitioners. The Flower Essence Society operates a Practitioner Referral Network, with a listing of about 3,000 flower essence therapists in the U.S. and Canada alone; contact Flower Essence Society, P.O. Box 459, Nevada City, CA 95959; tel: 530-265-9163 or 800-736-9222; website: www.flowersociety.org.

## The Soul Messages in Depression

While every person is different and the causes of depression are many, Patricia Kaminski has observed in her practice a common theme, or soul message, if you will. "I would say that the underlying emotional challenge is the inability to be in contact with deep feelings that have been somehow buried. When you work with a depressive person and you go deep enough into their biography, you will find a core level of grief, even a core level of anger, a core level of helplessness in some way."

The effect of burying a part of themselves is that they stop feeling. In contrast to the anxious person who feels too much, the depressive person isn't able to feel. Kaminski breaks down the word "depressed" into "deep-pressed," which is an accurate reflection of what is actually happening in this mood disturbance. "Something has been pressed down, a core level of response to life that should have been there, an emotion that should have been articulated—sometimes it goes back to childhood."

> **While every person is different and the causes of depression are many, Patricia Kaminski has observed in her practice a common theme, or soul message, if you will. "I would say that the underlying emotional challenge is the inability to be in contact with deep feelings that have been somehow buried."**

In response to this "deep-pressing," the soul gradually shuts down. Depression can be seen as the wisdom of the body, a stopping in one's tracks that is extreme enough to finally get the individual's attention. Kaminski likens it to a donkey who for some time has been abused, not fed well, neglected, and one day just lies down in the middle of the road and refuses to go any farther. The message of the donkey and of depression is: "I'm not getting back up until you take care of me and look at what's wrong with me." The analogy is apt for depression as the sufferer often can't get out of bed; the body just doesn't want to work anymore and the spirit has lost its love of life.

Antidepressants such as Prozac can serve as stimulants to get the body moving again, and in suicidal depression such intervention may be necessary to save a life. But from the flower essence perspective, truly dealing with depression involves identifying the core emotions that have been buried, "deep-pressed" in the person. In Kaminski's experience, the predominant emotion buried in men is commonly grief. In women, it's more likely to be anger, she says. This reflects our cultural belief and training that it is inappropriate for men to express grief and inappropriate for women to express anger.

Truly dealing with depression and other "mental" disorders through flower essence therapy also involves working in layers and is a process, not a quick fix, says Kaminski. "It's a whole developmental process for the soul. The developmental process involves steps . . . metamorphoses that have to happen. We have to work in a way to bring the consciousness up in the person. Whereas in typical medicine, what we do is mask the consciousness and stimulate the body in some way, what we do with flower essences is try to stimulate the consciousness to see these pictures, these parts of the soul."

The following case history reveals core emotions buried beneath a depression and demonstrates the layers of healing in flower essence therapy.

## Hank: Real Men Take Flower Essences

Hank, 40, had been suffering from depression for eight months and was on Zoloft when he came to Patricia Kaminski for help. The depression had started after his wife left him for a friend of his. Hank hadn't dealt emotionally with this doubly heavy blow. His attitude was to keep a stiff upper lip and tell himself, "I'm going to be okay. I'm pissed off at my wife, I'm pissed off at my friend, but so what, life goes on, big deal." His wife filed for divorce and took custody of their two children. His response was "Sure, you can have them, big deal." He didn't acknowledge how much it hurt to lose his children.

As time went on, Hank started drinking heavily and drinking alone; he had previously been a social drinker. He reported that he drank so he could sleep, and would often go to bed drunk, but then would wake up around three or four in the morning and not be able to fall back to sleep. He spent his time brooding and began to smoke more as well. He dated a little, but had so much anger at women that the dates didn't go well, and he concluded each time, "It's another bitch."

It was the situation at work that prompted Hank to go on Zoloft. He frequently arrived late, and his job performance had disintegrated. He had years of experience in construction, having started as a teenager, but now he was making a lot of mistakes. His coworkers were finding him difficult, describing him as hard to reach, sullen, moody, and lashing out at them for no reason.

About six months after his wife left him, his boss told him that even though he had worked for the company for many years, he couldn't keep him on unless Hank went through anger management or did something to clean up his act. Hank went to his doctor, who prescribed Zoloft.

The drug didn't do much for Hank, and he was wary of medication. When he had been on it for two months, a family friend who had been greatly helped by flower essence therapy suggested to Hank that there was another way to deal with what he was suffering from, which was depression. Hank hadn't put it together that that was what the Zoloft was for. Although he was very skeptical, he knew he needed to do something. With the high recommendation of the family friend, he decided to give it a try.

One of the reasons Patricia Kaminski chose this case to illustrate her work is that it is not the typical new age case that people often associate with this type of therapy. "A lot of times people think, flower essences, yeah, right, they're for flower fairies and freaks," Kaminski comments. But here was what you might call "a man's man," a hard-drinking, cigarette-smoking construction worker. While his case was not typical of Kaminski's depressive patients, in that his depression was not chronic, it illustrates how flower essence therapy can open the soul of someone who did not previously delve into the soul realm.

When Hank first came to her, Kaminski told him that it was up to him and his doctor to decide how to proceed with the Zoloft. She stressed that she is not a medical doctor and cannot tell someone to discontinue a drug. She did tell him, however, that as long as he was on the antidepressant, it was going to be a lot harder for her to get a clear emotional reading from him, and that was important because what they needed to work on was his feelings about what had happened to him.

She also shared with him her perception that the Zoloft was a crutch for him, and there was going to be a lot more strength for him in confronting these emotions. "I try to deal with where the person is in their life," explains Kaminski. "His thing was 'I'm a man, I can be on top of this, I'm not going to let it hurt me.' You want to appeal to what is noble about that. What is noble is that he wanted to be self-sufficient."

Hank didn't like the idea of being on Zoloft, having read about paranoia and other side effects associated with it. He also didn't want to be medicated. That was one of his reasons for seeking another approach. In the first month of flower essence therapy, he gradually went off the drug, but Kaminski was not involved in that process.

She started Hank right away on two flower essences, Gentian and St. John's wort, which she cites as good remedies for working with depression. "One of the reasons I used St. John's wort is that he looked so dark," explains Kaminski. "Of course he wasn't sleeping well, so he had dark circles under his eyes. You could just sense that the light was not in him, and his brooding quality, drinking, and smoking were signs of this."

It is important to note that the St. John's wort flower essence is distinct from the herbal remedy used for depression. The latter contains chemical components of the plant, while the former contains the *energetic* qualities. In this way, the flower essence addresses "the lack of light in the spiritual person, the anger, the brooding, the sullen quality. Even on a deeper level, with someone who needs St. John's wort, you sense that they're being sucked dry on a spiritual level. You could almost say, their shadow is getting all the juice.

"We have to remember that, just as we have physical parasites, we can attract psychic parasites, when we leave our soul wide open like that. When we have all that anger, and we're not dealing with it, there's a whole lot of beings in the universe that can feed off that. In a way, you can also say it's an infestation."

**For more about the concept of psychic parasites, see chapter 9.**

St. John's wort helps bring in light and also helps deal with irregular sleep patterns. Hank had reported that his sleep was disturbed by weird nightmarish dreams, which is another indication for this flower essence.

Gentian, the other remedy Kaminski gave to Hank, was developed by Dr. Bach. The indications for this remedy are when the soul has experienced a major setback and hasn't dealt with it; when the soul has reached a place where it seems nothing will help, and there is discouragement, almost cynicism. "It's a great remedy for the initial stages of depression because the soul has at some deep level given up, and the person is stuck," says Kaminski. This was the case with Hank. He had experienced a huge setback when the woman he had thought was his mate for life left him, and left him for a friend.

Hank took the flower essences every day, had appointments with Kaminski twice a month, and checked in with her at other times when he needed to. The first thing Hank noticed, during the first month of taking flower essences, was that he was sleeping better. Seeing that there was positive change gave him some confidence in the approach. The second thing that he noticed was that he was less moody on the job. His mood had lightened in general, he had better energy, wasn't as angry, and his work performance started to stabilize. By the end of the first month of treatment, he had gotten off Zoloft.

Then, one night three months after starting treatment, he went to a restaurant and saw his ex-wife and ex-friend there. "That was the turning point in therapy, from my point of view," says Kaminski. Whereas before such an encounter would have triggered anger in Hank, this time he felt deeply sad. He had to leave the restaurant. At home, he said he wanted to cry. He told himself, "I'm going to let myself cry, because no one's going to see me." As he told Kaminski later, "It hurt really damn bad" and felt like a knife in his heart.

Hank was ready for the next layer of healing. Kaminski had him stop taking his first two remedies and move to what she calls "heart remedies." First he took California Wild Rose. "It gives a lot of energy to the heart, but it helps the heart to feel the pain too," she explains. "It gives strength, but it helps to open the heart up. Roses have thorns. The package of love comes with pain. The heart has to start to feel that." Then after a month, she added Holly and Borage. "Borage is the remedy for the heart that helps most with the grief that the heart feels, and Holly, because we need to move to that place of forgiving others, and accepting."

Later, Kaminski added Bleeding Heart, which is specifically for the brokenheartedness of relationships. At the same time, she let Hank know that he needed to start dealing with the grief of losing his wife. "If your wife had died, you would grieve for her," she said. "She has died in a way, and you need to allow yourself to grieve for it."

Around this time, Hank started dating someone who turned out to be loving and able to be there for him. "That's one of the things about flower essences," says Kaminski. "It's not like they do everything for you, but they start changing the circumstances in your life, so that different things happen." Once that relationship started, she recalls, "you could almost see a whole other person. He was more relaxed. When he was seeing his kids on the weekend, he was having fun with them."

Kaminski gave Hank one final remedy, Yerba Santa, to help him look at his smoking. He was smoking a lot less, but wanted to quit completely. With the Yerba Santa, he got in touch with the grief at a core level in him. He shared with Kaminski that the grief he felt about his wife took him back to when his own parents got a divorce, when Hank was 12 years old. It was around that time that he smoked his first cigarettes, sneaking them from his father's pack. In the divorce, his two sisters went with his mother and he went with his father.

Hank had never before looked at the pain of his parents getting a divorce and the family being split up. He had never made the connection between that and taking up smoking. It was a breakthrough for him.

The final three months of his therapy with Kaminski were spent exploring his past and his current relationships, and revealing aspects of his soul life that he had never talked about before. As a result of this process, rather than simply blaming his wife, he came to see that he shared the responsibility for the failure of their marriage.

When Hank left treatment after six months, his depression, angry outbursts at work, and sleep problems had long since disappeared. He wasn't drinking much and that only socially.

He came back to Kaminski later for flower essences to support him during a stop-smoking program in which he had enrolled. She gave him Yerba Santa, Nicotiana, and Borage. He saw that smoking was another way that he was shutting down, "and that was the whole essence of his case, getting him to open up emotionally," she notes. "The more emotional empowerment occurred, the more ability he had to articulate his feelings, to be in touch with them and not be afraid of them, the more the depression broke up in him."

Hank's progress was aided by the fact that his depression was not a long-standing one and he had hardly been medicated at all, says Kaminski. "That's one of the strengths of flower essences. If we can get at the emotional patterns at a relatively early stage, flower essences show a good track record of helping. If someone has been depressed and medicated for years, it's a lot harder."

## The Medication of Souls

"It's not easy working with depression in our culture, because of the tremendous emphasis on medication," Kaminski states. "The longer somebody has been on psychiatric drugs, the more challenges we have. The sooner we can get to somebody, if they have been on the drugs for a short time, the more successful we're going to be. That's actually true of both flower essences and homeopathy."

It's not that people who have been on pharmaceuticals for a long time can't be helped by flower essences, it just makes the case more complex, she says. The flower essence practitioner has to work then with the chemical situation that has been set up in the body as well as with the emotional layers.

Kaminski cautions that this is not to say that people should simply throw away their antidepressants or other prescription drugs. Stopping needs to be done under the supervision of a qualified physician, and obviously if someone is psychotic or suicidal, the drugs may be saving his life.

Like Dr. Reichenberg-Ullman, Patricia Kaminski has a vision of another way that people can be helped in times of crisis. She would like to see doctors like the one who prescribed Zoloft for Hank put patients like him, whose depression was not life-threatening, on flower essences first. "That's what's happening in Cuba," she states. "The flower essences have become part of the medical model there. They've seen the results.

"What I would like to see is a revolution in the health-care industry, that at the early stages of intervention, when somebody needs emotional help, we provide, in addition to counseling, therapeutic modalities that are much safer and much more holistic. If those don't work, then we can consider stronger chemical options."

Again, with somebody who's psychotic or suicidal, immediate brain intervention in the form of medication may be necessary. "If your hand is in the fire, you can't go right to giving a remedy for healing the hand," says Kaminski. "The first thing you have to do is get the hand out of the fire." It's important to remember, however, that a tranquilizer or an antidepressant is never a cure, she cautions. Rather, it only temporarily changes behavior and enables the brain to function differently.

Unfortunately, those facts seem to have been forgotten. Kaminski points to an alarming trend in the use of pharmaceuticals. "It's just unconscionable to me how many people are being put on psychiatric drugs at the drop of a hat." Statistics on the huge increase in the prescription of such drugs over the past two decades demonstrate what Kaminski calls "the normalization of psychiatry."

In other words, she says, "more and more and more of the population are being medicated. If somebody comes in, suffering from lethargy, panic, anxiety, or PTSD [posttraumatic stress disorder], we right away medicate them. Children are being medicated. The elderly are being medicated. Prisoners are being medicated." What medication does is rob individuals of the capacity to deal with their soul and the messages it has to communicate, she says. "Whether it's conscious or unconscious, we're actually developing a model that is robbing people of their developmental capacity. There is a trend, both in psychiatry and in medicine, to medicate away problems."

The use of psychiatric drugs is behavior modification to help people adjust to their lives the way they are, according to Kaminski. "It isn't a transformative model of a human being. It's a behavioral adaptive model." She sees the results of this in people who come to her who have been on psychiatric drugs for a while—there is no movement in their lives.

The psychiatric drug model also seems to be promoting the idea that "we're supposed to somehow have the smiley face all the time," she observes. "The truth of the matter is, life hurts. There are failures and disappointments."

Kaminski envisions the development of a different model of human potential, one that doesn't only seek to fix, but asks why the breakdown happened. "What's standing in the way of that person being able to move on, to be a more loving and more productive person in human society? That for me is the goal of flower essence therapy—to wake people up, even if it's painful. When we open our heart to take risks, then our lives are more healthy, they're more whole."

# 8 Cellular Memory and the "Terrible Triad" of Depression: Soma Therapies

In the experience of Zannah Steiner, C.M.P., R.M.T., founder and clinic director of Soma Therapy Centre in Vancouver, British Columbia, depression typically involves both structural and emotional components. Addressing the structural aspect can effect significant changes in depression, but unless the emotional components are addressed as well, the structural balance may be thrown off again, "because we are body, mind, and spirit," explains Steiner. Addressing only one will not produce long-lasting benefits.

Steiner's expertise in the mind-body relationship stems not only from 20 years as a registered massage therapist, but also from a decade of study with osteopathic physician John Upledger, the originator of CranioSacral therapy and SomatoEmotional Release (see "Soma Therapies"). Through this work, she has gained a deep understanding of the relationship between emotional states and the body's structure. She founded Soma Therapy Centre to bring under one roof a variety of soma (body) therapies that she has found work well together to fully restore balance in the mind and body.

The body's structure refers mainly to bones, in particular, the bones at either pole of the craniosacral system: the sacrum (base of the spine) and the cranium (the skull). If these bones are out of alignment, the function of the craniosacral system can be thrown off, which affects the flow of the fluid that bathes the brain and spinal cord, called cerebrospinal fluid (CSF). Normally, CSF flows up and down the spine in a kind of rhythmic tide. When CSF is not flowing properly, it has a profound impact on the brain, nervous system, and entire body. (See "Soma Therapies" for a more detailed explanation of the craniosacral system.) Depression is one of many conditions that can result from structural misalignment and the attendant disturbed CSF flow.

"I think depression is oppression, repression, suppression, and compression," says Steiner. Contained in this statement are both the emotional and structural aspects of depression. Emotional trauma stored in the body is a reflection of oppression, repression, or suppression while structural distortion in the body produces compression. Compression is constriction due to pressure exerted on a body part or system. If the distortion is in the bones of the skull, for example, the result can be compression or a pressing on the brain and cranial nerves. Through soma therapies, these structural, functional, and emotional factors can be released and depression resolved.

## Depression's "Terrible Triad"

While every individual is unique and there is no depression template, the structural component frequently involved in depression is what Dr. Upledger termed "the terrible triad."

The terrible triad means a state of compression between the sacrum (base of the spine), the sphenoid (bone that, in part forms, the orbits of the eyes), and the occiput (the occipital bone, or back of the skull). In other words, these bone structures are producing constriction on the brain and dural membranes (the membranes covering the brain and spinal cord), and in the flow of CSF.

"In a case of depression or a case of chronic fatigue, we often discover that the sphenoid, the occiput, and the sacrum all seize up [become fixed, or immobile] at the same time," explains Steiner. This situation "gives us a clue that the person has compression on their brain and therefore a depressed nervous system function, and is likely suffering from some degree of emotional depression as well."

It is important to note at this point that the bones of the skull are not fixed, as many people believe. The skull "breathes" with the ebbing and flowing of the cerebrospinal fluid. Problems result when the bones become immobile due to misalignment, as is the case in the terrible triad under discussion.

In the skull, the temporal bones (the bones that the ears sit in) come together with the sphenoid and the occipital bones at flexible joints. The flexibility of these articulations between the skull bones is impeded when the temporal bones are in an asynchronous condition, meaning they are moving in opposition to each other with the ebb and flow of CSF, instead of together as they are meant to do. Asynchrony of the temporal bones sets the stage for the terrible triad and Steiner has found that it is often present with depression.

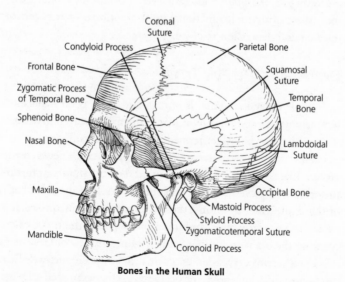

**Bones in the Human Skull**

The sphenoid, occipital, and temporal bones of the skull are involved in the "terrible triad" of depression.

When the temporal bones are not moving in synchrony, this restricts the normal movement of the bones of the head and the dural membranes, which transmits tension all the way down the spinal cord to the sacrum and reduces production and distribution of cerebrospinal fluid. The result is decreased mobility of the body in general and compromise of the immune and other systems, as CSF is vital to their operation. Thus rigidity and compression in the skull can have far-reaching neurological, functional, mental, and behavioral effects.

The terrible triad can result from a physical trauma such as a car accident, chronic injury, or systemic infection. Fortunately, CranioSacral therapy can release the compression in the craniosacral system and break up the terrible triad.

## Cellular Memory

An often overlooked source of depression is the body's storage of the emotions felt during traumatic events. Emotional residues are the basis of what is known as cellular memory. The body remembers all the traumas—whether physical injury or emotional upset—an individual has experienced because the attendant emotions are stored in its tissues. While psychotherapy can help uncover and make sense of many of the issues involved in the emotional component of depression, it may not effect their release from the body.

A trauma results in the formation of what Dr. Upledger termed "energy cysts" as the body walls off the trauma to store it locally, rather than allowing it to become systemic. Just as the body creates inflammation around the puncture site after you step on a nail, it forms an energy cyst in the body to contain the residues of strong emotions such as fear, anger, or resentment that remain in the body after a traumatic emotional event. For example, if as a child your mother looked at you with eyes like daggers, your body may have experienced it like a stab to the heart. The body then walled off the energetic residues in that area, creating an energy cyst in your chest, or the residues could be stored in muscles or organs somewhere else in the body. These energy cysts restrict the body's free flow of energy and movement, may produce discomfort, and become a localized source of dysfunction.[121]

Emotional residues can be stored in energy cysts anywhere in the body, including in organs. "The cellular memory in that energy cyst can be visual, kinesthetic [related to movement], auditory, or all of the above," Steiner explains. As the emotions are released from the energy cysts during SomatoEmotional Release (see "Soma Therapies"), patients reexperience the emotions and may remember the event involved. They may even assume the position they were in when the injury or trauma occurred.

As with all of the soma therapies, in SomatoEmotional Release the therapists take their cue from the patient's body. "We follow the body," explains Steiner, "If you were to feel in your own body the position that your body is inclined to go into, that would be the position that we would follow. Ultimately, it would take us to the injury that caused the position, so at the depths of that movement pattern is the original injury. You might have a memory of it. You might say, 'Oh, this is the fall from the tricycle at age three.'" Release can take place, however, even without the cognitive recall of the memory.

## Soma Therapies

The following techniques are the primary therapies used by Zannah Steiner and her colleagues at Soma Therapy Centre to address the structural, functional, and emotional components of depression and other disorders:

*CranioSacral therapy (CST):* This technique was developed by John Upledger, D.O., who defined CST as a "hands-on method of evaluating and enhancing the functioning of a physiological body system called the craniosacral system—comprised of the dural membranes and cerebrospinal fluid (CSF) that surround and protect the brain and spinal cord."[122] The word 'craniosacral' derives from the two poles of this system: the sacrum (base of the spine) and the cranium (the skull).

The skull is composed of interlocking bones that are far more mobile than most people think. Accident, injury, and the birth process can cause misalignment of the bone plates, resulting in what is termed cranial distortion. This distortion can in turn exert pressure on the brain (compression), impede the proper flow of CSF, and compromise the function of the nervous system.

The craniosacral system, which drives the flow of cerebrospinal fluid, operates as a semi-closed hydraulic pumping mechanism. "That pumping mechanism is responsible for ensuring that all of the fluids of the body are flowing," says Steiner. "Cerebrospinal fluid is the body's most important fluid. It is the basic 'soup stock' of the body, containing the ingredients—proteins, enzymes, and electrolytes—that are the basis of all other fluid systems." When CSF flow is diminished, fewer nutrients and less oxygen are delivered, and all other fluid systems are compromised. Thus, less CSF means less of everything else.

Compression in the skull and the attendant impeded CSF flow can produce symptoms throughout the body, from the more obvious, such as headaches and back pain to the less obvious, such as breathing and digestive disorders.[123]

## In Their Own Words

"Much of my body had seemed disconnected from me, but through . . . Somato Emotional Release, little by little, emotions were released from my body that my previous therapy was unable to do, and a deep soul purging came about, allowing my body to become connected again, and more than that, for my body and soul to become one. My whole being was emptied and yet left full. Full of feeling instead of numbness. Full of love instead of pain. Full of life instead of deadness . . . There was a wonderful releasing and letting go of the worthless chaff from my life's experiences, and I was left with the precious kernel of life, in its fullness and freeness. I was finally at peace with myself."

—a Soma Therapy patient

Examination using CST protocols (which include evaluation of the craniosacral system) determines the status of cerebrospinal fluid flow and nervous system function. By releasing restrictions in the craniosacral system through gentle manipulations, CST improves central nervous system function and has beneficial effects for many health conditons. According to the Upledger Institute in Palm Beach Gardens, Florida, these include central nervous system disorders, emotional difficulties, chronic fatigue, stress and tension-related problems, immune disorders, motor-coordination impairments, colic, autism, learning disabilities, fibromyalgia and other connective-tissue disorders, temporomandibular joint syndrome (TMJ), post-traumatic stress disorder, orthopedic problems, migraine headaches, and chronic neck and back pain.[124]

*SomatoEmotional Release (SER):* An offshoot of CST, SER is a hands-on technique developed around 1980 by Dr. Upledger and biophysicist Zvi Karni, Ph.D. SER works to aid the body in releasing the residual effects (energy cysts) of past traumas which can be emotional, viral, bacterial, or physical as from an injury or structural damage.

Through touch on areas where energy cysts are located, the therapist works with the patient's body-mind to release the emotional content of the blockages, relying on the messages communicated by the craniosacral system as a guide.

While some patients engage with the therapist in what is termed in SER "reflective dialogue technique," talking about what they are feeling in the process, the experience need not be articulated. It is as effective on a preverbal or nonverbal level, which makes SER an excellent method for releasing the residues of past traumas in infants and children.

The release of energy cysts often produces immediate emotional and physical benefits. As SER helps restore the free flow of energy and movement in the body, the conditions that can be ameliorated by the therapy may be limitless. Among those that Zannah Steiner cites as responding well are mental disorders, neurological disorders, chronic pain, whiplash, and degenerative diseases.

*Process-Oriented Counseling:* Also called Process Work, this is a therapeutic method developed by Jungian analyst Dr. Arnold

Mindell. It approaches areas of an individual's life that he or she experiences as "problematic or painful" and seeks to discover without judgment the meaning of and potential for personal growth contained in those areas. Symptoms in the body are "traced to their origin, whether they are of a physical, mental, emotional, and/or spiritual nature," Zannah Steiner explains. Process Work can aid CranioSacral therapy in effecting the release of emotional issues stored in the body.

*Visceral Manipulation:* This therapeutic technique for relieving restrictions and tensions in and around organs (viscera) was developed by French osteopath Jean-Pierre Barral in the early 1970s. "The basic philosophy of Visceral Manipulation is that an organ in good health has good movement," Zannah Steiner explains. When tissue becomes rigid or fixed, chronic irritation and dysfunction results. The function of surrounding tissue is also compromised as the tissue attempts to adapt to the change.

According to Dr. Barral, each organ in the body has its own biological rhythm, moving through five to eight cycles per minute. It actually moves subtly in a rotation around what Dr. Barral termed its own "embryogenic axis" or fulcrum, which is the orientation it had when the fetal organs were developing. Scar tissue from surgery or injury, chronic inflammation, or shortened fascia (fibrous connective tissue) can disturb the rhythm and suspension (rotation) of organs. Through specifically applied, light manual force, Visceral Manipulation releases the tensions and restrictions, and restores the proper mobility and inherent rhythm of the organs. As poor flow of cerebrospinal fluid can interfere with organ function, CranioSacral therapy is an important adjunct.

In addition to improved organ function, resulting benefits are better fluid circulation, relief of sphincter and muscle spasms, relief of chronic pain and tension, improved digestion and hormonal balance, and enhancement of localized and systemic immunity. "The organ system can be a storage facility of unexpressed emotion," says Steiner. "The organs are thought to contain the 'voice of the body.'" Thus, Visceral Manipulation can also release emotional holding. With the therapy, patients often experience a sense of well-being.[125]

**Resources** For information about CST, SER, and VM, contact the Upledger Institute/American CranioSacral Therapy Association, 11211 Prosperity Farms Road, Suite D-325, Palm Beach Gardens, FL 33410; tel: 561-622-4334; website: www.upledger.com. For CST, see the Canadian College of Osteopathy, Toronto, Ontario; website: www.osteopathy-canada.ca. For process-oriented counseling, see the website (www.aamindell.net) of Dr. Arnold Mindell, one of the founders of this type of therapy, or contact Process Work Center of Portland, 2049 NW Hoyt Street, Suite 1, Portland, OR 97209; tel: 503-223-8188; website: www.processwork.org.

## The Soma Approach

It's important to note that Steiner, like many natural medicine practitioners, does not rely on conventional diagnostic labels such as clinical depression to guide her treatment approach. "We do an assessment of each patient without knowing anything about their history," says Steiner. Treatment is then designed according to those presenting findings rather than being dictated by a label, symptom, or condition. Depression may be the indication for treatment, but there may be many other things happening in an individual that are causing it. Approaching a patient in this way allows for genuine treatment of that person at a deep level.

In addition, patients are viewed with new eyes at each visit, even if the visits are on consecutive days. This allows for adjustment in approach to changes that may have occurred as the result of the previous treatment or other factors. "We treat each patient as a completely new patient each time they come," says Steiner. "Otherwise, we'd be bringing an agenda or a bias into the treatment." This means that as a person moves through layers of healing, the therapy moves with her.

The approach Steiner has found most effective for soma therapies is an intensive week of therapy (two weeks is optimum), which means being treated five hours a day for five days in succession, predominantly with CST, Visceral Manipulation, and SER, but other therapies are used as needed. This program "bombards people's nervous systems to the point that they move through their issues in a week or two weeks," says Steiner. A "good percentage" of the Centre's patients (and likely a good percentage of the population at large as well) have suffered some form of abuse—whether physical, sexual, emotional, or spiritual abuse—and this intensive approach enables people to release their cellular memories of the abuse relatively quickly, emerge from crippling depression, and get on with the rest of their lives.

The following case illustrates how going through the body rather than primarily the mind can resolve emotional issues that verbal therapy may illuminate but often cannot quickly release.

## Leaving the Bed: Resolving Suicidal Depression

Karen, 39, suffered from suicidal depression and was taking "megadoses" of antidepressants (Elavil and Prozac), as she puts it. She had been on and off them since she was in her late twenties, and had been "very unhappy" for as long as she could remember. For three years prior to coming to Soma Therapy Centre, Karen had been experiencing terrible pain all through her body. "The only way I know how to describe it is knives slicing every inch, head to toe, 24 hours a day," she says. She also struggled with weight gain and chronic yeast infections.

In addition, she had mild but disconcerting seizures. She describes them as analogous to driving a car on the highway and suddenly putting it into neutral. "The car is still going and the wheels are still turning, but it's in neutral. All of a sudden my brain was not in motion." Karen was totally aware during these episodes, which lasted about 10 seconds, but could take no action. The seizures were erratic in occurrence. She would sometimes go quite a while without one, and then have as many as five a day.

For much of her adult life, Karen had no home; serving as a minister, she lived out of a suitcase and moved from place to place. When in her twenties she first began to seriously consider suicide, a woman she knew provided a "life raft" that Karen held onto through the years to come. "She helped me to promise myself that if I was on my bed, I was safe. Somehow that stuck, and so when I became suicidal, I always knew if I could just get to my bed, I wouldn't do anything." Although her surroundings were never the same, the bed wherever she was staying for the night became her safe place.

By the time Karen came to Soma Therapy Centre, however, the circumstances of her life had improved. She couldn't understand why she was still so depressed. "I was a minister, had a lot of love for people, and felt very fulfilled in what I was doing," she says. Before that she was a nurse, work she also loved doing. Further, she had spent many hours in therapy and filled thousands of journal pages in dealing with memories of sexual abuse that began to emerge eight years before she came to the Centre. "I had done a terrific job of working through my stuff. I did everything I knew how to do to move past it all. And yet, at some gut level, I just totally knew that it was still in there," says Karen.

A friend who had been greatly helped at the Centre tried to persuade Karen to go there. It took Karen a few years to agree because all the therapy she had undergone had left her depression intact. "I felt like I'd tried everything else and nothing had worked," she recalls. "Why would this be different? I was out thousands of dollars and my life was going downhill. Indeed, I was convinced I was not supposed to live past 40 years old. That was what the purpose of my life was: 40 years. I was really aware of dying. My body was shutting down."

Karen started with a mini-intensive. The therapies she underwent were CranioSacral therapy (of which SomatoEmotional Release is a component), Visceral Manipulation, and Process Oriented Counseling. She had treatment every day for three days in a row. "The first thing that happened," she remembers, "was I started feeling that deep core-level pain releasing. It felt like something was lifting off of me. Now I understand that my nervous system was decompressing. I had some really, really deep, painful treatments because my pain level was severe. To get it out you have to touch it, reach it." With the decompression of her nervous system, Karen's depression lifted, along with her body-wide pain. Zannah Steiner notes that Karen had the classic terrible triad described earlier in the chapter, which may have resulted from the abuse she had suffered.

In the process of treatment, Karen uncovered more memories of abuse. "There was a lot of emotional content, obviously, to my pain. Zannah would assess me and 'follow' my tissue. Most often that would take me to a position or pattern in my body, and as soon as I became aware, 'this is when such-and-such happened,' I would start to feel some release coming in my body. Then as I got the poignant details of how old I was, how many times it happened, or what belief system got put into place—all of those poignant details—I could feel my body releasing."

At first in treatment, Karen was dealing with the abuse she had worked on in her earlier verbal therapy. She felt it release from her body tissue. "It was different from the therapy I did before," she says. "Now I understood, 'That's why I feel the way I do. That's why I react the way I do. That's why I behave the way I do.'" After having CranioSacral therapy (with the SER component) and releasing the memories from her body tissue, the impact on her life wasn't apparent right away, aside from the lifting of the depression, Karen reports. But over time she began to see that she was reacting differently; she wasn't being triggered the way she used to be.

A few years after her initial treatment, Karen spontaneously got memories of her abuse as an infant, which she hadn't uncovered before. Before, such an occurrence would have plunged her into a depression, but it didn't. She signed on for a ten-day intensive at the Centre. "I had my worst seizure during that intensive," she recalls. "I actually almost passed out, kind of slid to the floor, and really touched bottom on it. I haven't had a seizure since."

That was two years ago now. Karen's body pain was alleviated in the middle of the first round of treatment and she went off antidepressants almost immediately. Her chronic yeast infection and weight problems have also been resolved. As for depression, "Zero," she says.

Today, Karen has a home and, having left the ministry, is now a CranioSacral therapist and Process Oriented counselor. At 44, she has survived the belief that her life was over at 40, and is thriving.

The lasting nature of the Soma Therapy treatment has been put to the test by recent emotional challenges, reports Karen. "I just lost my mother. With something like that before, I would have been in the depths of depression again. It's not just about having made some really positive changes in my life. I've really proven it to have held for me." In conclusion, Karen says, "I'm so set free. I got my life back. I think I get younger all the time now. If I can help somebody by telling about my experience, I would count it a privilege."

# 9 Trauma, Energy, and Spirit: Seemorg Matrix Work and Psychosomatic Medicine

When it comes to depression, "talk" therapy is a primary treatment (along with antidepressants) conventionally associated with the condition. While we have seen in this book that many factors that cause depression are not addressed by such therapy, we have also seen that psychospiritual issues frequently play a role and may need to be attended to for long-lasting resolution of the condition. This chapter explores two forms of psychotherapy that deal with the psychospiritual aspects of depression. The first, Seemorg Matrix Work, explores the interrelationship of trauma, energy, and spirit. The second, psychosomatic medicine, focuses on the effects of suppression of the spirit.

## Matrix Work

Tony Roffers, Ph.D., of Oakland, California, has been a psychotherapist for more than 30 years and has expertise in a range of psychotherapeutic techniques. Three years ago, he began using a method that results in such comprehensive healing for depression and other disorders that he now uses it as the centerpiece of his therapeutic practice. It is called Seemorg Matrix Work. Dr. Roffers works closely with the founder of the method, and aside from her is the most versed practitioner worldwide. Hundreds of therapists have been trained in this technique as word of its effectiveness has spread.

## What Is *Seemorg Matrix Work*?

Psychotherapist Asha Nahoma Clinton, L.C.S.W., Ph.D., developed Seemorg Matrix Work in the mid-1990s as a result of her dissatisfaction with the results produced by psychodynamic psychotherapy, which she had been practicing for 20 years. Matrix Work is "the first transpersonal, body-centered energy psychotherapy," to quote Dr. Clinton. "It treats trauma and its many psychological, physical, intellectual, and spiritual aftereffects with the movement of energy through the major energy centers."[126]

The transpersonal psychotherapy aspect of Seemorg Matrix Work is found in its focus on "removing the blocks that impede spiritual development" and "a spiritual technology to nurture and enhance that development."[127] Its name reflects this orientation; Simurgh, a fabulous bird featured in ancient Middle Eastern and Indian tales, is a symbol of the Divine.[128]

The major energy centers to which Dr. Clinton refers are the chakras, the series of seven energy vortexes positioned along the midline of the body from the base of the spine to the crown of the head. As discussed in chapter 3, when chakras are blocked, the free flow of energy in the body's field is impeded. Matrix Work uses the chakra system, progressing from top to bottom, to move negative energy out of the body. It then proceeds through the chakras from bottom to top, bringing positive energy into the body. This is the body-centered energy aspect of the therapy.

Dr. Roffers, who works closely with Dr. Clinton, explains the relevance of the chakras to psychotherapy: "The chakras are like switchboards for the meridian system, central energy centers for this electromagnetic circulatory system in the body. Seemorg Matrix Work is a way of working with your energy system that can put it back into alignment." According to Dr. Clinton's model, trauma is the source of aberrations in a person's energy field and those aberrations produce mind and body disorders.

There are essentially two kinds of traumas, says Dr. Roffers.

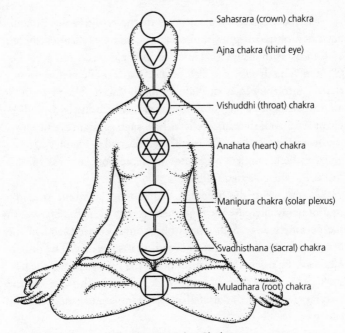

Sahasrara (crown) chakra

Ajna chakra (third eye)

Vishuddhi (throat) chakra

Anahata (heart) chakra

Manipura chakra (solar plexus)

Svadhisthana (sacral) chakra

Muladhara (root) chakra

The Seven Major Chakras

One is the crisis type of trauma, as in your father beat you or you fell off the garage roof. The other is developmental trauma, which is more subtle and occurs over a period of time. The experience of having a distant father or a critical mother is an example of developmental trauma. Dr. Clinton's therapy works with the energy system to clear those traumas in your body on an energetic level. With the traumas cleared and the energy balance restored, the disorders that stemmed from the energy aberration can self-correct.

The Matrix approach works in "a much more holistic, integrated way than the traditional talking therapy," states Dr. Roffers. It also significantly reduces the healing time, although it is still not a quick fix. "The metaphor I use is if you're going to remodel your kitchen and someone starts going into the walls and finds out where a leak is, pretty soon the whole kitchen may be torn apart."

133

Matrix Work can be effective in the traditionally difficult areas of multiple diagnosis, dissociation, and personality disorder, as well as with issues that are less complex, according to Dr. Clinton. The therapy can also be used to clear allergies, sensitivities, or intolerances as they are variously called. *Energy toxins* is another name for allergens (substances to which the body is allergic or sensitive); the name reflects how such substances can throw the energy system out of balance. As discussed in chapter 2, allergies can be an underlying factor in depression, as was true for Joshua, in the case that follows.

According to the Seemorg Matrix model, trauma is at the root of many allergies; the hypothesis is that the substance was in the person's energy field when the trauma occurred, and so the person developed "disharmony" with that substance. The disharmony can be reversed by reintroducing the substance into the person's field and using Matrix Work to move through all the chakras, removing the aftereffects of trauma and realigning the energy.

Dr. Roffers notes that regardless of how the allergy began, whether the hypothesis holds true or not, "aligning the meridians and the chakras in this way strengthens the person's system, aligns them, or puts them more in harmony with whatever the substance is." He adds, "I'm getting better results clearing energy toxins using Matrix Work, and specifically the clearing of traumas, than with any of the other methods I've used." Dr. Roffers is trained in several other energy-based allergy elimination techniques.

**Resources** **For information about Seemorg Matrix Work, contact Asha Nahoma Clinton, Ph.D., Energy Revolution, Inc., 885 East Road, Richmond, MA 01254; tel: 413-698-2191; office e-mail: MargieMatrix@aol.com; website: www.seemorgmatrixwork.com. The website has a directory of practitioners.**

## "Modern-Day Exorcism"

Dr. Roffers calls Matrix Work "modern-day exorcism." This is a reference to the legitimate and effective energy work that exorcism, as performed by skilled shamans of old, entailed (and still entails; see chapter 10). Matrix Work removes the energy influences to which we are subject today.

The work begins with the practitioner taking a thorough history, including what is known as a "trauma history." For the latter, clients list whatever traumas, of both the crisis and developmental types, they can remember.

To monitor the status of energy in the body throughout the work that follows, the therapist uses kinesiological muscle testing. For this, you hold one arm straight out in front of you and attempt to keep it there while the practitioner pushes down slightly on your arm. Normally, you can easily hold your arm in place, but when there is an energy disturbance in your meridian system, the muscle response is weakened. While you are being tested, the practitioner has you think of the trauma or asks you specific questions.

First, however, the practitioner tests you to make sure that you are not "neurologically disorganized." Other terms or phrases for this condition are "switched," being in "massive reversal," or having your polarization off, states Dr. Roffers. Regardless of the term, the upshot is that if you are in this state, muscle testing will not work on you.

To check for neurological disorganization, you place either hand on top of your head with the palm down, then extend your other arm out in front of you for the practitioner to test as in the standard muscle testing, Dr. Roffers explains. If the arm tests strong, the body is in alignment. When you turn the palm of the hand on your head up instead of down, the extended arm should test weak, because that position takes the body out of alignment. Any other combination (such as when the palm is down, the arm is weak; or when the palm is up, the arm is strong) is a reversal, a sign of neurological disorganization. The practitioner must then use a technique to realign the person so muscle testing will be accurate.

The next step in the Matrix process is the Covenant. The therapist starts by asking the client to say, "I give permission for my soul to be healed." If the arm response on that is weak, it means the person is not giving permission. "You have to clear that or they're not ready to be treated," Dr. Roffer states. "By clearing any negative beliefs that get in the way of treating traumas, the Covenant is a way of assuring that the person is going to be open to the treatment and, once you treat traumas, that those treatments will hold."

To clear the negative belief, you hold a hand over each chakra in turn, going from top to bottom, repeating the statement at each chakra. The therapist then conducts the muscle testing again to make sure that the negative statement has cleared from the body. A positive belief about the treatment (for example, "I can be healed") is then instilled in the same way, but by going up the chakras, from bottom to top.

While one hand moves from chakra to chakra, the other maintains a position over the primary chakra for that particular person, which is determined via muscle testing. The primary chakra is called the stationary point. Dr. Roffers observes that for many people it is the heart chakra, but it can be the solar plexus or another chakra. The client keeps one hand on the primary chakra throughout the process. "The two hands create an electromagnetic loop," he explains. "My hypothesis is that by closing that electromagnetic loop, you're realigning something in the body that's been misaligned and, as you clear that loop, something shifts. Then when you go to the next level, something else shifts." You will find that some chakras don't have any misalignment in them, he adds.

After the Covenant is completed, the therapist moves to clearing traumas, first identifying the primary chakra (stationary point) and a phrase that describes the trauma (for example, "My father abandoned me"). The client then moves down through the chakras, repeating the phrase at each.

There is no rigid order in proceeding with Seemorg Matrix Work, because it is tailored to the client, notes Dr. Roffers, but generally the focus at this point turns to the originating traumas.

These are the traumas that occurred very early in life. To clarify the nature of trauma, Dr. Clinton offers the following definition:

> A trauma is any occurrence which, when we think of it or it is triggered by some present event, evokes difficult emotions and/or physical symptoms, gives rise to negative beliefs, desire, fantasies, compulsions, obsessions, addictions or dissociation, blocks the development of positive qualities and spiritual connection, and fractures human wholeness.[129]

After working with the originating traumas, the focus shifts to the initiatory traumas, usually the events that brought the person into therapy. "These are the much more recent traumas," explains Dr. Roffers, "which are a retraumatization of the originating traumas."

Next step is to clear traumatic patterns. These are like a web of traumas that gets woven around an original trauma; you could also call this web a syndrome of traumas. For example, "if you had a very cold and distant father, you selectively attend to men who are that way, and you begin to attract men who are cold and distant, as a misguided attempt to heal," says Dr. Roffers. The belief, "All men are cold and distant," is formed secondarily and long after the originating trauma to which it is related.

*Another corollary of Seemorg Matrix Work is that it tends to open people up to spiritual possibilities. Clearing traumas and the self-sabotaging negative beliefs that cluster around them enable you "to become more whole within yourself, and you're much more open and permeable and interested in working on that spiritual level."*

The next step is to clear the negative or dysfunctional beliefs that have accrued as a result of traumas and instill the more positive or functional beliefs using the Core Belief Matrix. "A matrix is a cluster of interrelated core beliefs around a certain trauma," explains Dr. Roffers. A Core Belief Matrix is a series of statements, stated first in the negative and then in the positive, that reflect core beliefs. An example of a negative statement in a Matrix is "I can be used," while the corresponding positive statement is "I will no longer permit being used."

The client says each negative statement in turn, with the therapist conducting muscle testing. When a person says "I can be used" and the arm response is strong, it means the person believes that statement. Before proceeding to the next statement, "you have to take that dysfunctional belief out," says Dr. Roffers. The client goes down the chakras, saying the negative core belief. Then the corresponding positive core belief—"I will no longer permit being used"—is instilled by going up the chakras, repeating the positive statement at each chakra with one hand placed on the third-eye chakra (between the eyes) as the stationary point.

By clearing the traumas, traumatic patterns, and negative core beliefs and realigning the attendant energy imbalance, a condition such as depression can be resolved. As with other energy-based modalities, correcting the energy flow often results in self-correction of factors that present in depression and may seem to be the cause, such as neurotransmitter deficiencies.

As stated previously, another corollary of Seemorg Matrix Work is that it tends to open people up to spiritual possibilities. "To me, it's a major answer to how psychological work integrates with spiritual development," says Dr. Roffers. "If you have trauma, it separates you from God. It separates you from yourself. It separates you from others. It separates you from the Earth, the universe." Clearing traumas and the self-sabotaging negative beliefs that cluster around them enable you "to become more whole within yourself, and you're much more open and permeable and interested in working on that spiritual level." Having worked extensively with the Matrix method, he now believes that this clearing can be done for most people and for most types of trauma.

The following case history from Dr. Roffers' files demonstrates how Matrix Work can be used in combination with other therapeutic interventions to resolve depression.

distinct from organic disease in that diagnostics such as X rays, blood tests, and electrocardiograms can find none of the measurable changes of organic disease. In functional disease, the functions are being interfered with, but there is no sign of organic disease.

As an example of a psychosomatic disorder, Dr. Beckmann cites a 13-year-old girl who had not yet started to menstruate, but was beginning to look at boys. Her father, noticing this, told her that she should not look at any male aside from him until she was 16. When the girl still did not start menstruating in the next few years, her parents were concerned and took her to the doctor. The doctor determined that everything was fine; she did not have any organic disease that would interfere with menstruation. When she turned 16, released from "the program her father had impressed on her mind and psychic world," she began to menstruate. Freed from the conflict the prohibition posed to her, her body was free to become a woman.

## Conflict and the Spirit

In his practice, Dr. Beckmann deals with dilemmas of the mind, body, and spirit. (He notes that "the unconscious and the spirit are the same thing; one word in psychology, another in the religious sciences.") A conflict is at the root of all disorders, according to his model. Often, the conflict relates to childhood experiences. As a child, the person begins to suppress his own wishes, his own self, because when he shows his true self, it creates conflict with his father, mother, siblings, society. The threat of conflict trains the person into an adapted way of life, explains Dr. Beckman. "The person says, 'I cannot be myself because when I am myself I have problems with others.'"

At first, his spirit finds an outlet in dreams. As the conflict grows stronger, nightmares ensue. This reflects the mounting inner tension of suppressing the spirit, which can also be called the imaginary (imagination is a component of the imaginary). When dreams are remembered, that means the suppression is not complete. Nightmares are the spirit attempting to resolve the conflict and remove the blockage. When the nightmares stop, and dreams are no longer remembered, this means that the person has adapted to completely suppressing the conflict and to being "a good boy, a good student, the best." The price is suppression of his soul and his feelings.

This pattern is known as "the pathology of adaptation" or "the pathology of banality" because, without soul or spirit, life is banal, explains Dr. Beckmann. Although this example is about childhood, the same process occurs whenever the spirit is suppressed in order to "resolve" a conflict. It is not a true resolution, and body, mind, and spirit bear the consequences of the suppression. As in the Matrix model, internal conflicts that arise in adulthood are related to early childhood conflicts and their attendant messages, according to Dr. Beckmann.

"There is a law in nature that says you attract your similars," he says. "This is a law of chemistry and the same happens in the spiritual world," he says. If you have conflict and disorder internally, you attract conflicts that involve similar contradictions. This gives you the opportunity to resolve it this time and "get out of the disorder. We always attract what happens to us."

Dr. Beckmann adds that he believes even babies attract their similars. "They attract this terrible situation or this beautiful situation of family, of parents," he says. "They are not passive. They have an energy, a very powerful energy that attracts also." Viewed from this light, "you understand that the father and the mother are not the culprit or guilty party. This is not to exempt them from responsibility, because they could give the child a better life, but the real origin of the situation is in the person, in the laws of karma, in the direction of affinity."

## The Spirit's Message

In Dr. Beckmann's view, illness, whether depression or heart disease, arrives when "the development of the spirit has stopped or something that needs to happen is not happening. . . . We are not here to develop a body or psychology; these develop by nature. We are here to develop human consciousness, spirit—it's the same. To develop the behavioral virtues connected to this—to behave with wisdom, kindness, compassion, all the things that are related to love or justice, to purity, to connection with spirit."

Depression and other disorders, then, can be seen as the spirit's attempt to tell you something. Each form of response has its logic. Dr. Beckmann explains that the nature of the conflict dictates the manifestation. For example, physical symptoms relate to the stage of development during which the conflict originated. "Every organ or system in the body has its moment in the time loop. You would look at when the affected organ or system develops in the life of a child, then you would know when the conflict started."

In psychosomatic disorders, "the mind can't face the conflict and the imaginary helps to solve the conflict through the body in the form of functional disease." When the conflict is too great and the suppression is complete and goes on for too long, organic disease results. "Organic disease is the last development of the pathology of banality, of adaptation," says Dr. Beckmann.

In terms of "mental" disorders, the manifestation relates to the options contained in the conflict. In depression, the person waits for the solution to the internal conflict to come from outside, "doing nothing, staying there, waiting." In neuroses, such as obsessive-compulsive or anxiety disorders, the nature of the dilemma is that a solution exists, there are at least two choices and one of them offers a way out of the internal conflict, but the person doesn't act on it.

"This is the definition of neurotic," states Dr. Beckmann. "It is the conflict with the possibility of a solution, but the person stays in the continuous dilemma." An example is wanting to separate from a partner that you know, for your mental, physical, and spiritual well-being, you need to leave, and you have the financial and circumstantial wherewithal to do so, but you don't. In the case of one woman in this position, for years she thought to herself every day, "Soon I'll go." Then her husband had a stroke and half of his body was paralyzed. She could no longer play with the possibility of going, and now told herself, "I must stay. I now have no choice." The internal conflict was still there, however. With the continued suppression of her spirit, organic disease developed. Six months later, she had developed a brain tumor.

By contrast, in psychosis, there is no perceived way out of the conflict. Dr. Beckmann tells of a Russian woman who was brought to Spain by a man upon whom she was completely dependent (her pattern was dependence). He came home every night drunk and beat her. She could not go back to Russia, and she could not stay where she was. "This was a conflict that could only be solved through her mind. The only way to solve it was to go crazy." In psychoses, the imaginary has not been completely suppressed and is strong enough to provide an outlet through the mind.

One of Dr. Beckmann's patients experienced a trauma that, if her spirit had been suppressed, would have led to depression, anxiety attacks, or any other manifestation a spirit in distress might take. Instead, something different happened. This woman found out, after twenty years of marriage, that her husband had been cheating on her the whole time and had had lots of other women. She had thought all those years that she was the only one. "She was in shock after she found out," says Dr. Beckmann, "but she did not get ill because she said, 'Look, darling, you are very important, but for me the most important is God, life, energy, my relation to life.' She would not get ill because she had a higher connection and she had the right source. Her husband was not the source."

The woman in the case history that follows learned this lesson through a severe depression.

## Josephine: Reconnecting with the Spirit

Josephine, 38, had been severely depressed for a year and a half when she came to Dr. Beckmann. She had tried antidepressants, but they didn't help. She had two children, but had separated some time ago from her husband. Her depression began after she moved in with her boyfriend. She considered him her main problem. He was another child for her to take care of. He behaved like a two-year-old, stuck at the stage of what Dr. Beckmann calls "the little vandal." Addicted to cocaine, he took no responsibility in the household and brought no money home.

As things between them got worse and worse, her depression became more severe. The hormones in the birth control pill she was taking exacerbated her depression, so she stopped taking the pill, but the improvement was minor.

Josephine's conflict was that she had no money, her partner was not playing his part in the family, and "she had a vandal on her hands." This was not a new situation for her. Her husband and former boyfriends had been the same sort of man as her current mate. The depression was a new occurrence, however. In answer to why this was, given that she was playing out an old conflict, repeating a familiar pattern of disorder, Dr. Beckmann answers, "Because life gives you many possibilities. When you reach your limit, you need something stronger." In other words, the wake-up call from the spirit needed to be louder.

"From a spiritual point of view, she was unable to take a position

*Dr. Beckmann's method of approaching illness by looking for the internal conflict can produce quick results. In Josephine's case, she uncovered in their very first session the belief that she hadn't known she held. She saw that her dependency on men was creating the conflict behind her depression and understood the connection between that issue and her father. Two days after that first session, her depression lifted.*

to go, to make her own life, in her way, with her children," says Dr. Beckmann. Through working with him, Josephine learned that she held the belief, absorbed from her father, that she needed a man in order to exist. The internal conflict was that she had to stay with the man to exist, and yet existence with the man was terrible.

Dr. Beckmann's method of approaching illness by looking for the internal conflict can produce quick results. In Josephine's case, she uncovered in their very first session the belief that she hadn't known she held. She saw that her dependency on men was creating the conflict behind her depression and understood the connection between that issue and her father. Two days after that first session, her depression lifted.

The nature of spirit and internal conflict is illuminated by the fact that she didn't need to remove herself from the situation with "the little vandal" to gain relief. She was still living with him, he was the same person, and yet her depression disappeared. This is because she no longer had an internal conflict. She had brought into her consciousness the previously subconscious belief that she needed a man to exist, and she knew it wasn't true. Just knowing that dispelled the conflict.

"What I try to help my patients understand is that they will solve nothing by just going," says Dr. Beckmann. This is how the pattern was repeated in Josephine's life. Leaving one man only brought her to another of the same ilk because she hadn't dealt with the internal conflict and disorder that was attracting the similar to her again and again.

Josephine stayed in therapy with Dr. Beckmann to work on her issue of dependency. In his view, the issue would not be resolved until she connected with the spirit within, and felt a source of energy that did not rely on people or things for sustenance. The strength of that connection would enable her to do whatever it was she needed to do about her home situation.

Some people would say that this is simply a self-esteem issue, and Dr. Beckmann's reply is that self-esteem is a spiritual issue. "To have self-esteem you must have identity, and to find identity is to find the self. Finding the self leads you to spirituality."

## Marie: The Void Inside

"In this case, the person did not know who she was," says Dr. Beckmann, and the void inside of her led to deep depression.

Marie sought Dr. Beckmann's help when she was 32 years old. She told him, "I've lived my whole life without feeling and without suffering. I've never allowed myself to feel. I've never let myself be free. I've never loved a man. I've never felt pleasure." What she felt was apathy and a gaping emptiness.

She was severely depressed, but had avoided antidepressants. For the past five years, she had been living with a man she didn't love. When he went to work in the morning, she would go back to bed and stay there until right before he came home. When he did, she told him all the things she had done with her day, all of it made up. She couldn't tell him that she couldn't work, couldn't do anything, in fact.

Recently, the man had begun saying that they should get married and have children. While they were vacationing in Spain, Marie "made an escape" and came to Dr. Beckmann. The present conflict was clear: he wanted to marry; she didn't, and she had never loved anybody. In the course of the session, it emerged that Marie's mother and father hadn't loved each other when they got married, and despite the fact that their marriage had remained loveless, they were still married and living together.

But Dr. Beckmann and Marie did not begin to get to the real issue behind her depression until he said, "You act like a little girl. What happened with your mother?" Marie said, "She's impossible. She's always treating me like a little girl." Suddenly she stopped and then amended her statement, "No, my mother acts with me like a little girl." She revealed that her mother even spoke to her like a little girl who cannot talk very well.

In Marie's case, Dr. Beckmann asked the mother and father to meet with him in separate sessions. He discovered that Marie's mother was in love with her own father, Marie's grandfather. He was a very good man. Marie's mother loved him dearly, as a girl loves a good father. At seven years old, she was separated from her family, sent to live with an aunt in a faraway city. She didn't know why. She cried herself to sleep every night and dreamt about her father. A year and a half passed, and then she was sent back to her family. Restored to the arms of her father, Marie's mother took up her happy childhood again.

Sitting in Dr. Beckmann's office, at the age of 64, Marie's mother realized that she had never asked why she was sent away as a child. After that, she set about discovering the reason. All it took was asking her older brother. He explained that in that period their family was in dire economic straits, and they sent her to the aunt who was better off.

The separation had grave consequences for Marie's mother. She married a man she didn't love. Two months before her first child (Marie) was born, her father died. "It was like the end for her," said Dr. Beckman. She wanted to die so she could be with him. But at the same time, there was this beginning in the form of a baby. Marie's mother told Dr. Beckmann that in the first moment she saw Marie's face, she saw the face of her father. "I imagined myself to be dead like my father," she said. "I imagined my daughter and I dying. I would have exchanged my daughter for my father."

At that moment, in the mother's eyes, "the baby changed into the father," says Dr. Beckmann. And from that point on, Marie lived a life that was not her own; she lived her life in her mother's life. "Ever after the daughter lived an empty existence. She didn't know where the emptiness and the terrible depression were coming from. She told me, 'I'm crazy. I cannot live anymore.'"

In this case, the fact that she didn't know who she was was not Marie's problem, but her mother's problem. Her mother had taken her life from her. For Marie, the resolution of her depression took longer than it did for Josephine. At the end of three months of treatment, Dr. Beckmann brought mother and daughter together in a session. Marie's mother told her in her own words what she had done. She sobbed and told Marie how sorry she was. With her mother's acknowledgement of what had happened and her confirmation that Marie had good reason for the emptiness she had felt all her life, the depression began to clear.

Marie did not marry the man she did not love, although both her mother and father wanted her to. She left him and moved to Spain. After a period of hostility toward her parents, she restored amicable relations with them. "She is making her way alone and is not depressed anymore," says Dr. Beckmann. "The first time she began to feel, she was newborn. Now she is a person who feels and is so happy about it that she is even happy to feel the sadness that comes sometimes. There's no more emptiness."

# 10 Shamanic and Psychic Healing

While shamanic practice and psychic healing may seem to be in a completely different category from the other therapies covered in this book, they are actually not far from those discussed in the previous chapter and others throughout that address issues of the mind and spirit. They each have their own ways of dealing with these issues in depression and other disorders, but the goal is the same: the clearing of negative influences and blockages, and the restoration of balance, wholeness, and connectedness.

The negative influences and blockages addressed by shamanic and psychic healing are found in the energy field that surrounds the body, which is also called the aura. While, unlike shamans and psychics, laypeople cannot typically see their aura, they receive evidence of its existence all the time. Have you ever "felt your skin crawl" when you met someone new? Have you ever suddenly and for no apparent reason felt drained or depressed when you walked into a room of people? These reactions are the result of discordant foreign energies entering your energy field, or aura, where they are not a good match with your energy and consequently produce a sense of unease or discomfort.

Unfortunately, energy influences are not just transitory. The energy field around your body is subtle and fragile and can actually be damaged, which renders it more permeable to foreign energies and more likely that they will remain. Among the events or practices that can damage or pollute the aura are emotional or physical trauma, psychic or verbal abuse, other people's negative or bad thoughts about you, and substance abuse. Physicians and psychics alike have noted that the energy field can be poisoned or polluted by harmful energies that produce mental, emotional, and physical symptoms and, if allowed to remain, can lead to disease.[130]

Psychiatrist Shakuntala Modi, M.D., of Wheeling, West Virginia, has been researching energy field disturbances for over 15 years. She has identified a range of physical and psychological symptoms and conditions that result from such disturbances, including depression, headaches, allergies, uterine disorders, weight gain, stammering, panic disorders, and schizophrenia. Further, under clinical hypnotherapy, 77 out of 100 patients cited foreign "beings" in their aura as responsible for the symptoms or condition for which they were pursuing treatment. Dr. Modi's research revealed that these beings are "the most common cause of depression" and "the single leading cause of psychiatric problems in general."[131]

Dr. Modi also found that after removing the foreign energies from the patient's energy field using hypnotherapy, the patient's symptoms "often cleared up immediately."[132]

The concept of energy disturbances in a person's energy field causing a variety of physical and psychological problems is gaining greater recognition and acceptance in the healing professions and among the public at large. A simple way to look at the issue of "energy pollution" is that, like the environment and your body, your energy field is subject to toxic buildup and requires cleansing to restore it to health. Just as we take measures to clean up our planet and engage in various body detoxification methods such as fasts or colonics, we need to take steps to clear the toxins from our auras. Shamanic and psychic healing are methods for cleansing your energy field of the toxins that are interfering with your physical, emotional, and spiritual health.

## Shamanic Healing

Shamanism is "perhaps the oldest form of practical spirituality in the world, originating in the time of Ice Age people, going back as far as 35,000 B.C."[133] It is also practiced virtually everywhere in the world. A shaman is someone who has gone through advanced initiation into the "hidden" realm. The shaman uses the knowledge gained for healing and the good of the community. Shamanic healing is psychic healing. The terms are separated in this chapter to delineate indigenous shamanic practice from psychic healing that is not rooted in traditional ritual.

Malidoma Patrice Somé, Ph.D., is an internationally celebrated African shaman, diviner, and teacher who brings the healing wisdom of the Dagara tribe to the West. Dagara country is an area situated at the intersection of Ghana, the Ivory Coast, and Burkina Faso (formerly Upper Volta) in western Africa. Dr. Somé left his homeland to study in Europe and the United States and holds three master's degrees and two doctorates from the Sorbonne and Brandeis University. He has authored two books, *Ritual: Power, Healing, and Community* and *Of Water and the Spirit.*

The latter is his moving autobiography, which tells of his kidnap at the age of four by Jesuit missionaries who kept him prisoner and trained him as a missionary until at twenty he managed to escape. After an arduous trip back to his village, he underwent an initiation that restored him to his people and opened the way to his shamanic practice. While conducting workshops and classes around the world, Dr. Somé maintains close connection with his village in Burkina Faso.

One of the things Dr. Somé encountered when he first came to the United States in 1980 for graduate study was how this country deals with mental illness. When a fellow student was sent to a mental institute due to "nervous depression," Dr. Somé went to visit him.

"I was so shocked. That was the first time I was brought face to face with what is done here to people exhibiting the same symptoms I've seen in my village." What struck Dr. Somé was that the attention given to such symptoms was based on pathology, on the idea that the condition is something that needs to stop. This was in complete opposition to the way his culture views such a situation. As he looked around the stark ward at the patients, some in straitjackets, some zoned out on medications, others screaming, he observed to himself, "So this is how the healers who are attempting to be born are treated in this culture. What a loss! What a loss that a person who is finally being aligned with a power from the other world is just being wasted."

On the ward, Dr. Somé also saw a lot of "beings" hanging around the patients, entities that are invisible to most people but which he was able to see. "They were causing the crisis in these people," he says. It appeared to him that these beings were trying to get the medications and their effects out of the bodies of the people the beings were trying to merge with, and were increasing the patients' pain in the process. "The beings were acting almost like some kind of excavator in the energy field of the people. They were really fierce about that. The people they were doing that to were just screaming and yelling." He couldn't stay in that environment and had to leave.

Mental disorders are spiritual emergencies, spiritual crises, and need to be regarded as such, says Dr. Somé. The Dagara people view these crises as "good news from the other world." The person going through the crisis has been chosen as a medium for a message to the community that needs to be communicated from the spirit realm. The community helps the person reconcile the energies of both worlds—"the world of the spirit that he or she is merged with, and the village and community."

That person is able then to serve as a bridge between the worlds and help the living with information and healing they need. Thus, the spiritual crisis ends with the birth of another healer. "The other world's relationship with our world is one of sponsorship," Dr. Somé explains. "More often than not, the knowledge and skills that arise from this kind of merger is a knowledge or a skill that is provided directly from the other world."

The beings who were increasing the pain of the inmates on the mental hospital ward were actually attempting to merge with the inmates in order to get messages through to this world. The people they had chosen to merge with were getting no assistance in learning how to be a bridge between the worlds, and the beings' attempts to merge were thwarted. The result was the sustaining of the initial disorder of energy and the aborting of the birth of a healer.

"The Western culture has consistently ignored the birth of the healer," states Dr. Somé. "Consequently, there will be a tendency from the other world to keep trying as many people as possible in an attempt to get somebody's attention. They have to try harder." The spirits are drawn to people whose senses have not been anesthetized. "The sensitivity is pretty much read as an invitation to come in," he notes.

Those who develop so-called mental disorders are those who are sensitive, which is viewed in Western culture as oversensitivity. Indigenous cultures don't see it that way and, as a result, sensitive people don't experience themselves as overly sensitive. In the West, "it is the overload of the culture they're in that is just wrecking them," observes Dr. Somé. The frenetic pace, the bombardment of the senses, and the violent energy that characterize Western culture can overwhelm sensitive people.

## Depression and Purpose

With depression, anxiety, and addiction, which are virtual epidemics in the United States, Dr. Somé has found that the main underlying problem is disconnection from one's life purpose. This disconnection "leaves room for some alien energies to come in that don't have anything to do with the kind of promise the person made before coming into this world," the promise of what one will fulfill in one's life. "When you make a promise like that, and you come here and you start doing something else, you're subject to depression." With this come feelings of uselessness or helplessness, a sense of being "completely adrift in a world without purpose."

The shaman can see what a person's purpose is. "The divination doesn't hide these kinds of things," says Dr. Somé. The shaman's task in this case is to tell people their purpose, but only after preparing them through ritual so they are in a position to understand what is revealed. The ritual used is called a "dupulo," and works to correct the changes done to the original promise.

"It's like a disruption of the current path the person is in, which is depression. It prepares the space for the promise to come alive in the person." After the ritual, the shaman lets a week or two pass, to let it sink in, and then helps the person to become consciously aware of their promise, the specifics of their purpose.

At that point, it is up to them to "take it or leave it," Dr. Somé says. "If they decide to not fulfill that purpose, they'll find themselves back in depression." The choice is theirs—they can choose to be depressed or choose to be aligned with their path.

Dr. Somé gives the example of a man whose promise before being born, the reason why he came into this world, was to work at providing homes for people. "That's a metaphor for a variety of things. One is the actual physical home, another is helping people to feel comfortable with themselves. The man shows up here, finds out how difficult it is, and winds up working in a factory." After receiving the information about his purpose, "he can either start looking into the possibility of being a home-builder or a healer who brings stability or groundedness to other people, or not."

## Longing for Connection

Another common thread that Dr. Somé has noticed in depression and other "mental" disorders is "a very ancient ancestral energy that has been placed in stasis, that finally is coming out in the person." His job then is to trace it back, to go back in time to discover what that spirit is. In most cases, the spirit is connected to nature, especially with mountains or big rivers, he says.

In the case of mountains, as an example to explain the phenomenon, "it's a spirit of the mountain that is walking side by side with the person and, as a result, creating a time-space distortion that is affecting the person caught in it." What is needed is a merger or alignment of the two energies, "so the person and the mountain spirit become one." Again, the shaman conducts a specific ritual to bring about this alignment.

Dr. Somé believes that he encounters this situation so often in the United States because "most of the fabric of this country is made up of the energy of the machine, and the result of that is the disconnection and the severing of the past. You can run from the past, but you can't hide from it." The ancestral spirit of the natural world comes visiting. "It's not so much what the spirit wants as it is what the person wants," he says. "The spirit sees in us a call for something grand, something that will make life meaningful, and so the spirit is responding to that."

That call, which we don't even know we are making, reflects "a strong longing for a profound connection, a connection that transcends materialism and possession of things and moves into a tangible cosmic dimension. Most of this longing is unconscious, but for spirits, conscious or unconscious doesn't make any difference." They respond to either.

As part of the ritual to merge the mountain and human energy, those who are receiving the "mountain energy" are sent to a mountain area of their choice, where they pick up a stone that calls to them. They bring that stone back for the rest of the ritual and then keep it as a companion; some even carry it around with them. "The presence of the stone does a lot in tuning the perceptive ability of the person," notes Dr. Somé. "They receive all kinds of information that they can make use of, so it's like they get some tangible guidance from the other world as to how to live their life."

When it is the "river energy," those being called go to the river and, after speaking to the river spirit, find a water stone to bring back for the same kind of ritual as with the mountain spirit.

"People think something extraordinary must be done in an extraordinary situation like this," he says. That's not usually the case. Sometimes it is as simple as carrying a stone.

## Rituals for the West

One of the gifts a shaman can bring to the Western world is to help people rediscover ritual, which is so sadly lacking. "The abandonment of ritual can be devastating. From the spiritual viewpoint, ritual is inevitable and necessary if one is to live," Dr. Somé writes in *Ritual: Power, Healing, and Community.* "To say that ritual is needed in the industrialized world is an understatement. We have seen in my own people that it is probably impossible to live a sane life without it."[134]

Dr. Somé did not feel that the rituals from his traditional village could simply be transferred to the West, so over his years of shamanic work here, he has designed rituals that meet the very different needs of this culture. Although the rituals change according to the individual or the group involved, he finds that there is a need for certain rituals in general.

One of these involves helping people discover that their distress is coming from the fact that they are "called by beings from the other world to cooperate with them in doing healing work." Ritual allows them to move out of the distress and accept that calling.

Another ritual need relates to initiation. In indigenous cultures all over the world, young people are initiated into adulthood when they reach a certain age. The lack of such initiation in the West is part of the crisis that people are in here, says Dr. Somé. He urges communities to bring together "the creative juices of people who have had this kind of experience, in an attempt to come up with some kind of an alternative ritual that would at least begin to put a dent in this kind of crisis."

Another ritual that repeatedly speaks to the needs of those coming to him for help entails making a bonfire, and then putting into the bonfire "items that are symbolic of issues carried inside the individuals. . . . It might be the issues of anger and frustration against an ancestor who has left a legacy of murder and enslavement or anything, things that the descendant has to live with," he explains. "If these are approached as things that are blocking the human imagination, the person's life purpose, and even the person's view of life as something that can improve, then it makes sense to begin thinking in terms of how to turn that blockage into a roadway that can lead to something more creative and more fulfilling."

The example of issues with an ancestor touches on rituals designed by Dr. Somé that address a serious dysfunction in Western society and in the process "trigger enlightenment" in participants. These are ancestral rituals, and the dysfunction they are aimed at is the mass turning-of-the-back on ancestors. Some of the spirits trying to come through, as described earlier, may be "ancestors who want to merge with a descendant in an attempt to heal what they weren't able to do while in their physical body."

"Unless the relationship between the living and the dead is in balance, chaos ensues," he says. "The Dagara believe that, if such an imbalance exists, it is the duty of the living to heal their ancestors. If these ancestors are not healed, their sick energy will haunt the souls and psyches of those who are responsible for helping them."[135] The rituals focus on healing the relationship with our ancestors, both specific issues of an individual ancestor and the larger cultural issues contained in our past. Dr. Somé has seen extraordinary healing occur at these rituals.

Taking a sacred ritual approach to depression and other disturbances rather than regarding the person as a pathological case gives the person affected—and indeed the community at large—the opportunity to begin looking at it from that vantage point too, which leads to "a whole plethora of opportunities and ritual initiative that can be very, very beneficial to everyone present," states Dr. Somé.

## Healing and Belonging

With shamanic healing, as with any other kind of healing, there needs to be an agreement with the recipients that they are indeed willing to heal. "There's a lot of resistance to healing," comments Dr. Somé. "There's more of an acceptance of the pathology as a means of getting attention than there is a desire to get out of there." He cites the societal isolationism or tendency to be alone in your own space as one of the contributing factors to this pattern. Illness is one path to a sense of belonging.

"We have to understand that there is in the human being a certain instinct towards belonging. When that doesn't happen, the creative self goes to heavy-duty work to try to figure out all kinds of different ways to belong. Pathology can become a very cozy area of belonging, and people will hang onto their own pain because that's what makes them feel alive."

Dr. Somé helps open people's eyes to another kind of belonging. It doesn't happen overnight, but there is "a gradual emergence in the person of a certain perception of themselves and of the world that makes them gradually realize that they do fit, that in fact, the way they used to feel has shifted from a pathology to a healership." They see that they actually have a gift that can benefit people.

With this realization, they enter a completely different arena of belonging. They are now part of the group that has something to give to the world. "Giving is a very tangible form of belonging," says Dr. Somé. This approach is a powerful way of turning depression around. "The reorientation of the person away from isolation into a sense of collective belonging transcends dramatically the feeling of being useless."

While Dr. Somé's tradition of shamanic healing has its roots in West Africa, its addressing of energetic influences and occupation of one's energy field by foreign entities or "beings" is similar to the focus of psychic healing.

## Psychic Healing

Psychic healing involves the removal of foreign energy from your energy field, says Reverend Leon S. LeGant, of San Rafael, California. He has been a clairvoyant all his life and has worked as a psychic healer for the past eight years, clearing hundreds of people of the disruptive influences in their energy fields. Now, as executive director of the Psychic School, a nonprofit organization dedicated to the development of psychic abilities, he is devoting much of his time to training others in this type of healing.

Simply put, a psychic is someone who is sensitive to nonphysical forces. LeGant believes that everyone is psychic to some degree. Their abilities vary depending on when they shut themselves down, which most people do between the ages of three and five in response to parental and societal invalidation of the spirit realm, he says.

LeGant defines clairvoyance as "the ability to see energy in the form of mental image pictures. Since everything in the universe is made of energy, you can see it clairvoyantly in the form of a symbol or image or a picture that would make sense to the person seeing the information or the image." He notes that, without the proper context for the visions, clairvoyance is easily labeled hallucination.

Childhood fears of the dark, of monsters in the closet, of things under the bed actually have foundation in reality, arising as they do from children's "clairvoyance sensing an energy in the room with them." Since it is frightening, they begin to turn off their clairvoyance, explains LeGant. The programming of the educational system and, usually, their parents supports this suppression. "There's no validation for clairvoyance or being sensitive," he notes.

The imaginary friends of childhood also indicate children's connection to the spirit realm. These friends are their spirit guides. Again, messages from outside invalidate what children know to be true and teach them that "what they're sensing and seeing is not real, it's just an illusion or something they're making up." In most families, growing up requires that you stop having tea with your imaginary friends.

For some people, suppressing contact with the spirit realm is more difficult than for others. Psychics actually have "slightly different neurochemistry," LeGant explains. "Their pineal gland is usually a little larger, and there may be a genetic component to it that affects their brain chemistry and allows them to process energy in the form of images and thoughts in their mind." In adolescence, the brain chemistry shifts, and the clairvoyance becomes highly active again. It takes that amount of time for the body to develop and be able to receive the information. Around the time that the neurochemistry changes is when psychics become hypersensitive. They can easily be overwhelmed by everything they are taking in and all that they are feeling as a result. "It's a lot to process," says LeGant, who speaks from personal experience.

A "grounded psychic" can balance between the physical and spiritual worlds and distinguish them from each other, but few psychics are assisted in accomplishing this until they are adults and are fortunate enough to find the help they need in handling their abilities. This has implications for mental disorders. While you as a depressed person may not identify as a psychic, at the very least you share with psychics the characteristic of hypersensitivity.

## The Psychic Aspects of Depression

Anyone with a mental illness is being influenced on some level through their spiritual sensitivity, says LeGant. In the case of depression, most who suffer from it are highly sensitive people. "They get overwhelmed with other people's emotions, other people's problems, other people's pain. They often get cut off from their own emotions because they're flooded with everyone else's. Foreign energy gets absorbed into their body, into their aura, into their chakra system, and becomes a very heavy, weighted energy." Being overwhelmed in this way can lead to both depression and anxiety.

> *Anyone with a mental illness is being influenced on some level through their spiritual sensitivity, says Leon LeGant. In the case of depression, most who suffer from it are highly sensitive people. "They get overwhelmed with other people's emotions, other people's problems, other people's pain. They often get cut off from their own emotions because they're flooded with everyone else's."*

Becoming overwhelmed by foreign energy is especially likely to happen to healers. Psychotherapists, doctors, spiritual healers, and others in the healing profession "may not know how to handle another person's energy, so they end up absorbing their pain and their problems. . . . If they're absorbing someone else's problem into their space, that problem will start to attract matching problems to them in their own life. Then they're trying to solve that problem, but it was never their problem in the first place." Frustration, confusion, and eventually depression typically result.

Pain is stuck energy, and when you absorb it, it weighs you down. "Someone who gets that overwhelmed and flooded with foreign energy leaves their body," says LeGant. Regardless of the fact that the mind has checked out and is no longer aware of the foreign energy, the body continues to absorb others' pain (stuck energy) and its own energy flow becomes blocked. "An antidepressant helps in the sense that it shuts down the person's clairvoyance and sensitivity and they feel less overwhelmed, but the pain is still in their body." This is why after many people go off antidepressants and the chemical leaves their system, they become overwhelmed again. "It's because the pain's still there," he says.

## The Beings in Your Energy Field

In addition to feeling overwhelmed, another component of depression in the psychic model is spirit attachment. To understand how this works, it is necessary to consider life forms in the dimensions beyond the third dimension in which we live.

"Fifth dimensional life forms are angels and the various beings of the angelic hierarchy. The fifth dimension is what most religions and forms of spirituality would consider heaven," explains LeGant. "The fourth dimension is the in-between world where lost souls go if they are disconnected from the Supreme Being or confused. For example, someone who has died and is in resistance toward leaving their family and moving on will be in this dimension."

The fourth dimension, which intersects our world, is home to a lot of beings, which are energy life forms that could also be called spirits. There's a wide spectrum of beings, whose nature depends upon their evolution, LeGant says. "Some are just observers, just watching and not interfering, some are very nice, helpful healers, and some are very destructive, harmful, negative beings that will lead people into mental illness, from suicide to depression to schizophrenia." They lead people into many other places as well. There's a being for almost everything, according to LeGant, and the influence of their dark energy is responsible for the negative state of the world.

There are beings that feed on sexual crime, on war, on negative thoughts, on control, on punishment, and on specific kinds of illness. "The more common beings in depression are 'punishment beings,' 'victim beings,' and 'hopelessness beings,'" he says, although the beings present depend entirely upon the individual. Depressed people are also often influenced by "oppression beings" that push them down every time they try to find enthusiasm, excitement, or joy.

LeGant knows about these beings through his "reading" of hundreds of people in the course of his work as a psychic healer. Over the years, he has repeatedly encountered these different types of beings in clients' energy fields. Note that the destructive beings LeGant identifies are different from the beings Dr. Somé observed in the mental institute, which were occupying the patients' energy fields to help them become healers.

The thoughts and emotions that depressed people experience have a lot to do with the beings in their space. The mechanism behind the transmittal of thoughts is the fact that we all are telepathic, meaning we can pick up on others' thoughts. For example, you might be excited about changing your life in some way, and then you get this foreign thought telling you, "You can't do this, you'll fail, it's not going to work, it's hopeless, it's useless." That is the being in your space talking to you. "If it's a really nasty being, like a 'suicide being,' it will say, 'It's so hopeless, you may as well kill yourself, that's what you need to do,' and then the person is in so much pain that that's what ends up happening," says LeGant. "Those thoughts can be very intense and quite overwhelming."

The problem is that most people don't realize that these are not their thoughts, and they think that this is how they feel. People who are not developed clairvoyantly can't see the negative energy, so it is able to influence them and create confusion and angst. Influence by a being is often the case in people who go from doctor to doctor, or other healer, looking for a solution to their problem, to no avail. "What they need is someone to help them move the beings out of their space," LeGant says, and this is what a spiritual healer such as he does.

## Pain Ridges and Core Pictures

In order to attach to people, the beings need something to anchor into. That something is pain, in the form of pain ridges and core pictures within people.

Pain ridges are energy blockages in the body that are formed during traumatic experiences. The pain associated with that trauma is stored in the body as a block of emotional energy, a pain ridge. "The beings plug into those pain ridges, into that old emotional energy, and it's like twisting a knife in someone's back," says LeGant. "They stimulate the old energies so the person continues to experience, or sits, in old emotion that has nothing to do with what's going on in present time."

Beings also attach to what are called "core pictures." These are made up of the emotions, thoughts, and sensory information associated with a trauma and are stored in the subconscious. Naturally, the content of core pictures is unique to each individual but, as with the beings that are present, LeGant has seen common themes to the core pictures in the many depressed clients who have come to him. In general, these pictures tend to be those of invalidation, punishment, and hopelessness. Other common categories are apathy pictures, death pictures, and suicide pictures. The core pictures provide another anchor for beings who feed on that type of energy. The beings then keep that old energy strong—"lit up," as LeGant refers to it.

Some of the pain ridges and core pictures are from past life-times, and are often the result of past-life suicides. Suicide beings stimulate these past-life death ridges and pictures, which contain the thoughts, emotions, and concepts of that long-ago moment of suicide. The body is always in present time, however, so it experiences the replaying of this pain as though it is happening now. "When the body gets stuck in a death picture, it will feel like it's dying," says LeGant. "It will experience what went on in that life-time and there's no rational explanation for where that emotion or that fear is coming from."

Again, prescription medications will numb people to the painful reenactment of their core pictures, but the pictures are still there.

As the previous discussion illustrates, the feeling that depressed people have of being overwhelmed arises from more than the circumstances of their lives or the exhaustion and deple-tion that accompany depression. With the flood of foreign energy from other people and occupation by negative beings that con-tinually restimulate painful experiences and support the feelings of helplessness and uselessness associated with depression, it is no wonder they feel overwhelmed.

## Spiritual Healing

LeGant prefers to call what he does "spiritual healing" rather than "psychic healing" because the former is a more accurate description of what he is in fact doing, which is clearing the blockages to a person's connection to Spirit. He refers to this higher power as "the Supreme Being," which reflects its primacy over all the destructive beings that can occupy your energy field. A strong connection to the Supreme Being is your best protection against the negative beings, who cannot thrive in an atmosphere of Light.

Spiritual healing involves erasing the core pictures, removing the pain ridges, and clearing all the negative beings from the person's space. Again, the content of all of this is unique to the individual, so the healing is never the same from one person to the next. In a session, LeGant and the client sit across from each other in comfortable chairs. To do his work, he goes into a light trance and, with eyes closed, "reads" what is happening in the client and sets about clearing the energy. Clients can choose to close their eyes or not during the process. By its very nature, psychic work does not require the client to be present; spiritual healing can also be done over the phone, which is how LeGant works most of the time.

LeGant has found depression one of the easiest of the "mental disorders" to clear, and so his success rate with depressed clients is high. People who have become addicted to the depression, however, may try to take themselves back into it, even after clearing, he says. "Some people have been in it for so long that the thought of coming out of it is frightening to them." As Dr. Somé pointed out, it is comfortable and familiar. "There's a level of safety there. They can stay home and not have to deal with certain things." When they try to return to their depression after spiritual healing, they often discover that, with the energetic impetus for it gone, they can't quite achieve it.

Some people become scared by feeling good after the energy that kept their depression in place is removed. Feeling good "lights up another layer of pictures for them." These might be from when they were children and got punished when they were too exuberant. A core picture formed around the belief that when they are feeling joyful, something bad is going to happen. In that case, the pictures and beings that make it uncomfortable for them to be happy need to be removed.

It is also necessary for people with depression to learn how to handle their sensitivity, so they will not go back to absorbing the pain, emotions, and problems of people around them, says LeGant, who himself suffered from depression for years. More specifically, his message to those who are depressed is that you need to learn how to "be senior to energy" and how to define your own reality. This means not letting the beings or others' energy determine your reality. His experiences in coming to understand his sensitivity, learning the mechanics of depression, and discovering what worked to heal himself are part of the reason he is so successful in clearing depression in his clients.

Leon LeGant is a graduate of the Berkeley Psychic Institute (BPI). There are many psychic healers; for help in choosing one, you may want to contact BPI or a similar institution for a recommendation. Berkeley Psychic Institute, Berkeley, CA; tel: 510-548-8020; website: www.berkeleypsychic.com. Lisa French, one of LeGant's teachers, does psychic healings as described in this chapter. She now runs the Clairvoyant Center of Hawaii; tel: 808-328-0747 or 808-329-ROSE (7673); website: www.magicisle.com/reading.htm

## Celia: 20 Years of Occupation

Celia, 65, had suffered from severe, debilitating depression for 20 years. She had checked herself into mental hospitals three times over that period due to suicidal impulses. She had tried numerous antidepressants and various forms of therapy, but nothing alleviated her condition.

A registered nurse specializing in psychiatrist nursing, and later a therapist, Celia had not been able to work much since her depression began. She would try at different times, but each time had to give it up. Finally, she got a job overseeing a board-and-care home. Someone else ran it, and all she had to do was paper-work. She was also supposed to check on the place once a week, but the most she could manage was once every two months. She barely left her bedroom and was in a constant state of apathy.

It took three sessions with LeGant to lift Celia out of her depression. In the first round, he cleared a lot of beings that were suppressing her and beating her up in an energetic sense. There were "punishment beings," "oppression beings," "self-trashing beings" that would get her to trash herself, "apathy beings," "hopelessness beings," and "suicide beings." There were also "a few fallen angels, which are pretty vicious," he says.

He also cleared the core pictures that the various beings were "feeding" on, and discovered that there were core pictures actually programming her to be depressed. "She had been in the depression for so long that core pictures had developed around that, containing information that this is the way to be, this is how you handle things." He had to remove those first, and then underneath found "a lot of original family programming from childhood." The main theme in these core pictures was invalidation. Celia had had a tyrannical mother who yelled and was verbally abusive. There were quite a few layers of childhood pictures that LeGant had to remove.

"She was asleep in the chair the whole time I was working on her," he recalls. "She couldn't be in her body when I was dealing with that level of pain, which is unique. I don't see that too often."

After the first session, her depression got worse, which LeGant had warned her would happen. "I pulled the core pictures out. Those are like the keystones in an arch. When you pull the keystones out, a lot of stuff starts falling apart. Some people have built their life on their pain. You go in and take out that foundation and everything starts to go into flux; they redefine their reality. In the process of that, things die, and the person can feel as if they're dying or like things are falling apart. In her case, a lot of pain poured out of her body."

LeGant calls this a growth period. The first week after the first session is usually very intense, he notes. "After a week it starts to lighten up. After two weeks, you start to notice the joy underneath. It starts to come in and replace the pain with more lightness. If someone's in a crisis with their growth period, I just let them know that they can contact me. Usually they just need reassurance that it's normal. They don't need me to do anything."

In Celia's case, he gave her a month to recover between the first and second sessions. He felt she needed that amount of time "to catch up and release everything associated with what I had pulled out." The next two sessions dealt with clearing another level, the next layer, of beings. "There were more core pictures around childhood and failure, and around taking a career [nursing] that was not her career, but was her parents' wanting her to do something, which was not validating in the long run for her." As a therapist, she had also absorbed a lot of people's pain, and that energy needed to be cleared.

Celia was not so overwhelmed after the second session and, after the third, her depression lifted. In the period that followed, a lot of problems in her life—financial and household issues—began solving themselves. "Initially after she came out of it, she would want to go into it, but couldn't," says LeGant. "There was a level of safety in being numb and being able to hide under the covers. She would try to do it, but she couldn't make it for more than three to four days." Then she stopped being able to go into the depression at all.

When Celia would get hit by some news within the family, an emotional family matter to which before she would have responded by climbing into bed and being depressed, now she would just take a nap and then get on with the activities of her day. As for work, she has retired from nursing and, given her propensity to absorb others' energies, she has decided not to resume work as a therapist. She is exploring pursuits that will be a better fit for her and, therefore, validating of the changes she has made.

# Appendix B
## Resources

*Practitioners in this book*

**Johannes Beckmann, M.D., Master of Psychosomatic Medicine**
Clínica Paracelsus Mallorca
Calle Francisco Vidal Sureda, 23
E-07015 Palma de Mallorca
Spain
Tel: 34 971 70 28 00
Fax: 34 971 40 13 16
E-mail: johanbe@terra.es

Dr. Beckmann is the medical director of the sister clinic to Dr. Rau's Paracelsus Klinik in Switzerland (see Dr. Rau's listing below). The medical practice is similar, being based in biological medicine, with the addition of psychosomatic medicine, which is Dr. Beckmann's specialty.

**Ira J. Golchehreh, L.Ac., O.M.D.**
2175-D Francisco Blvd.
San Rafael, CA 94901
Tel: (415) 484-4411

Licensed as an acupuncturist, doctor of oriental medicine, doctor of alternative medicine, and qualified medical evaluator (Q.M.E.) for the State of California, Dr. Golchehreh runs a general practice specializing in internal and external disorders, pain-related disorders, and sports/orthopedic medicine.

**Patricia Kaminski**
Flower Essence Society
P.O. Box 459
Nevada City, CA 95959
Tel: (800) 736-9222 (U.S. & Canada) or (530) 265-9163
Fax: (530) 265-0584
E-mail: pkaminski@flowersociety.org
Web site: www.flowersociety.org

Patricia Kaminski is an herbalist, flower essence therapist, co-director of the Flower Essence Society, author of *Flowers that Heal*, and co-author of *Flower Essence Repertory.*

The Flower Essence Society is an international membership organization of health practitioners, researchers, students, and others interested in deepening knowledge of flower essence therapy. FES is devoted to research and education, and offers training and certification programs, and publications. The Society also provides a free networking service for finding a practitioner in your area.

**Dietrich Klinghardt, M.D., Ph.D.**
1200 112th Avenue NE, Suite A100
Bellevue, WA 98004
Tel: (425) 688-8818

Dr. Klinghardt specializes in Neural Therapy, Applied Psychoneurobiology, and Family Systems Therapy to address the transgenerational energy legacies at the root of illness.

**Rev. Leon S. LeGant**
Tel: (415) 459-4585
E-mail: leon@psychicschool.com
Website: www.psychicschool.com

Rev. LeGant is a psychic clairvoyant, spiritual healer, and executive director of the Psychic School, a nonprofit organization dedicated to the development of psychic abilities, spiritual awareness, and self-healing. The school offers readings, classes, retreats, short- and long-term training programs, and long-distance spiritual education.

**Thomas M. Rau, M.D.**
Paracelsus Klinik Lustmühle
CH-9062 Lustmühle b. St. Gallen
Switzerland
Tel: 41 71 335 7171
Fax: 41 71 335 7100

E-mail: dr.thomas.rau@paracelsus.ch
Website: www.paracelsus.ch

The Paracelsus Klinik is a center for European biological medicine and holistic dentistry. All chronic diseases are treated in this clinic, where medical doctors and dentists work together under one roof. The Klinik has a branch in Palma de Mallorca, Spain, directed by Dr. Johannes Beckmann (see page 175).

**Judyth Reichenberg-Ullman, N.D., L.C.S.W.**
The Northwest Center for Homeopathic Medicine
131 Third Avenue North
Edmonds, WA 98020
Tel: (425) 774-5599
Website: www.healthyhomeopathy.com

In practice with her husband, Robert Ullman, Dr. Reichenberg-Ullman is a licensed naturopathic physician board certified in homeopathy. She has been practicing for 18 years and is the author/co-author of six books on homeopathic medicine, including *Prozac Free, Ritalin-Free Kids,* and *Whole Woman Homeopathy.*

**Tony Roffers, Ph.D.**
P.O. Box 27463
Oakland, CA 94602
Tel: (510) 531-6730
E-mail: tonyroffers@earthlink.net

Dr. Roffers is a licensed psychologist whose private practice with adult clients emphasizes Thought Field Therapy and Seemorg Matrix Work for a wide variety of problems including depression, anxiety, panic disorder, PTSD, addiction, and food and inhalant sensitivities.

**Malidoma Patrice Somé, Ph.D.**
236 West East Avenue, Suite A, PMB 199
Chico, CA 95926
Tel: (530) 894-0740
E-mail: rowenap@jps.net (Rowena Pantaleon, Dr. Somé's assistant)
Website: www.malidoma.com and www.villagewisdom.net

Dr. Somé is an African shaman, diviner, and teacher who brings the healing wisdom of the Dagara tribe to the West.

**Zannah Steiner, C.M.P., R.M.T.**
Soma Therapy Centre
2607 West 16th Avenue
Vancouver, BC V6K 3C2 Canada
Tel: (604) 731-7883
E-mail: soma@intouch.bc.ca
Website: www.somatherapy.info

The Centre offers a range of Soma (body) therapies, particularly utilizing CranioSacral therapy, Visceral Manipulation, and SomatoEmotional Release to address the root causes of a disorder. Other therapies include acupuncture, chiropractic, psychological counseling, massage, and hydrotherapy. Among the conditions commonly treated are depression, chronic fatigue, immune deficiencies, chronic pain, paralysis, addictions, autism, developmental delays, and ADD.

**Bradford S. Weeks, M.D.**
P.O. Box 740
Clinton, WA 98236
Tel: (360) 341-2303
E-mail: admin@weeksmd.com
Website: www.weeksmd.com

Dr. Weeks' medical and psychiatric orientation is biological and biochemical, with a particular focus on anthroposophic medicine. Among the therapeutic modalities he employs in this context are targeted nutritional therapies, IV therapies for detoxification and replenishment, apitherapy (bee venom therapy), and Psychology of Mind. In his practice, he treats people with dis-ease of all kinds, from "mental" disorders to severe degenerative physical disorders such as multiple sclerosis, arthritis, immune dysfunction, cardiac disease, and cancer. He always looks for the reasons that the patient feels they are ill and how the patient wants to change things once wellness is reclaimed. A favorite question for patients is: What are you doing with your creative energy?

# Endnotes

## Introduction

1. C. J. L. Murray and A. D. Lopez, eds., "Summary: The Global Burden of Disease: A Comprehensive Assessment of Mortality and Disability from Diseases, Injuries, and Risk Factors in 1990 and Projected to 2020" (Cambridge: Harvard School of Public Health on Behalf of the World Health Organization and the World Bank, Harvard University Press, 1996). Available on the Internet at: http://www.who.int/msa/mnh/ems/dalys/intro.htm. Cited in U.S. Department of Health and Human Services, "Mental health: A report of the Surgeon General, Executive Summary," (Rockville, Md.: U.S. Department of Health and Human Services, Substance Abuse and Mental Health Services Administration, Center for Mental Health Services, National Institutes of Health, National Institute of Mental Health, 1999), ix.

2. Ibid.

3. R. C. Kessler, et al., "A Methodology for Estimating the 12-Month Prevalence of Serious Mental Illness," in: *Mental Health, United States, 1999*, ed. R. W. Manderscheid and M. J. Henderson (Rockville, Md.: Center for Mental Health Services, 1998), 99–109.

4. Center for Mental Health Services, *Survey of Mental Health Organizations and General Mental Health Services* (Rockville, Md.: Center for Mental Health Services, 1998).

5. D. P. Rice and L. S. Miller, "The Economic Burden of Schizophrenia: Conceptual and Methodological Issues, and Cost Estimates,"

in *Handbook of Mental Health Economics and Health Policy: Schizophrenia*, ed. M. Moscarelli, A. Rupp, and N. Sartorious, vol. 1 (New York: John Wiley and Sons, 1996), 321–4.

6. The full text of the letter is available on the Internet at: http://www.connix.com/~narpa/mosher.htm

## 1 What Is Depression?

7. Ronald Hoffman, "Beyond Prozac: Natural Therapies for Anxiety and Depression," *Innovation: The Health Letter of FAIM* (January 31, 1999), 10–11, 13, 15, 17, 19.

8. Bradford Weeks, M.D., "Mental Health," available on the Internet at: www.weeksmd.com/articles/mental.html.

9. Bika Reed, *Rebel in the Soul: A Dialogue Between Doubt and Mystical Knowledge* (Rochester, Vt.: Inner Traditions International, 1987).

10. Thanks for this idea goes to: Demitri Papolos, M.D., and Janice Papolos, *Overcoming Depression: The Definitive Resource for Patients and Families Who Live with Depression and Manic-Depression* (New York: HarperPerennial, 1997), 10.

11. P. Stokes and A. Holtz, "Fluoxetine Tenth Anniversary Update: The Progress Continues," *Clinical Therapeutics* 19:5 (1997), 1135–250.

12. National DMDA, "Consumer's Guide to Depression and Manic Depression," National DMDA (Depressive and Manic-Depressive Association), 730 North Franklin Street, Suite 501, Chicago, IL 60610-3526; tel: (800) 826-3632 or (312) 642-0049; website: http://www.ndmda.org.

13. Ibid.

14. Quoted in: Demitri Papolos, M.D., and Janice Papolos, *Overcoming Depression: The Definitive Resource for Patients and Families Who Live with Depression and Manic-Depression* (New York: HarperPerennial, 1997), 10.

15. *The Global Burden of Disease: A Comprehensive Assessment of Mortality and Disability from Diseases, Injuries, and Risk Factors in 1990 and Projected to 2020* ed. C. Murray and A. Lopez (Cambridge: Harvard University Press, 1996).

16. NARSAD (National Alliance for Research on Schizophrenia and Depression), Research, "Conquering Depression," NARSAD

Research, 60 Cutter Mill Road, Suite 404, Great Neck, NY 11021; tel: (516) 829-0091; fax: (516) 487-6930; website: www.narsad.org.

17. Ibid., "Fact Sheet: The Warning Signs of Suicide."

18. NAMI, "Understanding Major Depression," NAMI (National Alliance for the Mentally Ill), Colonial Place Three, 2107 Wilson Blvd., Suite 300, Alexandria, Va. 22201-3042; tel: (888) 999-NAMI (6264) or (703) 524-7600; website: www.nami.org.

19. NARSAD, "Fact Sheet: The Warning Signs of Suicide," NARSAD (National Alliance for Research on Schizophrenia and Depression), 60 Cutter Mill Road, Suite 404, Great Neck, NY 11021; tel: (516) 829-0091; fax: (516) 487-6930; website: www.narsad.org.

20. Demitri Papolos, Md., and Janice Papolos, *Overcoming Depression: The Definitive Resource for Patients and Families Who Live with Depression and Manic-Depression* (New York: HarperPerennial, 1997), 10.

21. C. Brown and H.C. Schulberg, "Diagnosis and Treatment of Depression in Primary Medical Care Practice: The Application of Research Findings to Clinical Practice," *JMPT (Journal of Manipulative & Physiological Therapeutics)* 21:7 (September 30, 1998), 504.

22. American Psychiatric Association, "Practice Guideline for Major Depressive Disorder in Adults," *American Journal of Psychiatry* 150:4 supplement (1993). M. Olson and H. Pincus, "Outpatient Psychotherapy in the U.S.: Volume, Costs, and User Characteristics," *American Journal of Psychiatry* 151 (1994), 1281–8.

23. Harvard Medical School, "Update on Mood Disorders: Part II," *Harvard Mental Health Letter* 11:7 (1995), 3.

24. "Depression Drugs Widely Prescribed to Children," *Health Watch* 4:2 (June 30, 1999), 2.

25. American Psychiatric Association, *DSM-IV-TR (Diagnostic and Statistical Manual of Mental Disorders, 4th Edition, Text Revision)*, Washington, DC: American Psychiatric Association, 2000: 345.

26. Ibid., p. 356.

27. National DMDA, "Consumer's Guide to Depression and Manic Depression," National DMDA (Depressive and Manic-Depressive Association), 730 North Franklin Street, Suite 501,

Chicago, IL 60610-3526; tel: (800) 826-3632 or (312) 642-0049; website: www.ndmda.org. Demitri Papolos, M.D., and Janice Papolos, *Overcoming Depression: The Definitive Resource for Patients and Families Who Live with Depression and Manic-Depression* (New York: HarperPerennial, 1997), 4.

28. Lewis Wolpert, *Malignant Sadness: The Anatomy of Depression* (New York: The Free Press, 1999), vii, 1.

29. Ronald Hoffman, "Beyond Prozac: Natural Therapies for Anxiety and Depression," *Innovation: The Health Letter of FAIM* (January 31, 1999), 10–11, 13, 15, 17, 19.

30. NARSAD, "Fact Sheet: The Warning Signs of Suicide," NARSAD (National Alliance for Research on Schizophrenia and Depression), 60 Cutter Mill Road, Suite 404, Great Neck, NY 11021; tel: (516) 829-0091; fax: (516) 487-6930; website: www.narsad.org.

31. Rita Elkins, *Depression and Natural Medicine: A Nutritional Approach to Depression and Mood Swings* (Pleasant Grove, Utah: Woodland Publishing, 1995), 16. Demitri Papolos, M.D., and Janice Papolos, *Overcoming Depression: The Definitive Resource for Patients and Families Who Live with Depression and Manic-Depression* (New York: HarperPerennial, 1997), 270.

32. Catherine Carrigan, *Healing Depression: A Holistic Guide* (New York: Marlowe and Company, 2000), 7.

33. Lewis Wolpert, *Malignant Sadness: The Anatomy of Depression* (New York: The Free Press, 1999), 3–4.

34. Ibid, 5–6.

35. Demitri Papolos, M.D., and Janice Papolos, *Overcoming Depression: The Definitive Resource for Patients and Families Who Live with Depression and Manic-Depression* (New York: HarperPerennial, 1997), 32–3.

36. Catherine Carrigan, *Healing Depression: A Holistic Guide* (New York: Marlowe and Company, 2000), 75.

37. Joseph Glenmullen, M.D., *Prozac Backlash* (New York: Touchstone/Simon & Schuster, 2000), 16.

38. E. C. Azmitia and P. M. Whitaker-Azmitia, "Awakening the Sleeping Giant: Anatomy and Plasticity of the Brain Serotonergic System," *Journal of Clinical Psychiatry* 52:12 suppl. (1991), 4–16.

Cited in Joseph Glenmullen, M.D., *Prozac Backlash* (New York: Touchstone/Simon & Schuster, 2000), 16.

39. Joseph Glenmullen, M.D., *Prozac Backlash* (New York: Touchstone/Simon & Schuster, 2000), 340.

40. *Taber's Cyclopedic Medical Dictionary*, 17th ed. (Philadelphia: F. A. Davis Company, 1993), 662, 1318.

41. Joseph Glenmullen, M.D., *Prozac Backlash* (New York: Touchstone/Simon & Schuster, 2000), 16.

42. Michael T. Murray, N.D., *Natural Alternatives to Prozac* (New York: Quill/William Morrow, 1996), 4.

43. Ibid., 2.

44. Ibid., 2.

45. Maryann Napoli, "A New Assessment of Depression Drugs," *HealthFacts* 24:7 (July 31, 1999), 4.

46. C. Pande and M. E. Sayler, "Adverse Events and Treatment Discontinuations in Fluoxetine Clinical Trials," *International Journal of Psychopharmacology* 8 (1993), 267–9.

47. Peter R. Breggin, M.D., and David Cohen, Ph.D., *Your Drug May Be Your Problem: How and Why to Stop Taking Psychiatric Medications* (Reading, Mass.: Perseus Books, 1999), 68.

48. Joseph Glenmullen, M.D., *Prozac Backlash* (New York: Touchstone/Simon & Schuster, 2000). Peter R. Breggin, M.D., and David Cohen, Ph.D., *Your Drug May Be Your Problem: How and Why to Stop Taking Psychiatric Medications* (Reading, Mass.: Perseus Books, 1999), 46–7

## 2: Sixteen Causes of Depression

49. Rita Elkins, *Depression and Natural Medicine: A Nutritional Approach to Depression and Mood Swings* (Pleasant Grove, Utah: Woodland Publishing, 1995), 8.

50. Richard Leviton, *The Healthy Living Space,* (Charlottesville, Va.: Hampton Roads, 2001) 2.

51. Ibid., 3.

52. "Doctors Warn Developmental Disabilities Epidemic from Toxins," *LDA (Learning Disabilities Association of America) Newsbriefs* 35:4 (July/August 2000), 3–5; executive summary from the report by the Greater Boston Physicians for Social Responsibility,

*In Harm's Way—Toxic Threats to Child Development,* available at http://www.igc.org/psr/ihw.htm; for LDA, http://www.ldanatl.org.

53. Philip J. Landrigan, *Environmental Neurotoxicology,* (Washington, DC: National Academy Press, 1992) 2; cited in Richard Leviton, *The Healthy Living Space,* (Charlottesville, Va.: Hampton Roads, 2001), 13.

54. Cited in: Syd Baumel, *Dealing with Depression Naturally* (Los Angeles: Keats Publishing, 2000), 31.

55. Sherry A. Rogers, M.D., *Depression—Cured at Last!* (Sarasota, Fla.: SK Publishing, 1997), 94.

56. John Foster, M.D., "Is Depression Natural in an Un-natural World?" *Well-Being Journal* (Spring 2001), 11; website: www.wellbeingjournal.com.

57. Catherine Carrigan, *Healing Depression: A Holistic Guide* (New York: Marlowe and Company, 2000), 62.

58. Syd Baumel, *Dealing with Depression Naturally* (Los Angeles: Keats Publishing, 2000), 34–7.

59. Dietrich Klinghardt, M.D., Ph.D., "Amalgam/Mercury Detox as a Treatment for Chronic Viral, Bacterial, and Fungal Illnesses," lecture presented at the Annual Meeting of the International and American Academy of Clinical Nutrition, San Diego, September 1996.

60. Morton Walker, D.P.M., *Elements of Danger: Protect Yourself Against the Hazards of Modern Dentistry* (Charlottesville, Va.: Hampton Roads, 2000), 138, 141.

61. Ibid., 144–5.

62. Syd Baumel, *Dealing with Depression Naturally* (Los Angeles: Keats Publishing, 2000), 34.

63. Ibid., 35.

64. W. D. Kaehny, et al., "Gastrointestinal Absorption of Aluminum from Aluminum-Containing Antacids," *New England Journal of Medicine* 296 (1977), 1389–90. D. P. Perl and A. R. Bordy, "Detection of Aluminum by Semi-X-Ray Spectrometry with Neurofibrillary Tangle-Bearing Neurons of Alzheimer's Disease," *Neurotox* (1990), 133–7. Morton Walker, D.P.M., *Elements of Danger: Protect Yourself Against the Hazards of Modern Dentistry* (Charlottesville, Va.: Hampton Roads, 2000), 218–9.

65. Sherry A. Rogers, M.D., *Depression—Cured at Last!* (Sarasota, Fla.: SK Publishing, 1997), 165–7.

66. Ibid., 166.

67. Personal communication, 2001.

68. Rita Elkins, *Depression and Natural Medicine: A Nutritional Approach to Depression and Mood Swings* (Pleasant Grove, Utah: Woodland Publishing, 1995), 117.

69. Sherry A. Rogers, M.D., *Depression—Cured at Last!* (Sarasota, Fla.: SK Publishing, 1997), 460.

70. Ibid., 461–2.

71. John N. Hathcock, *Nutritional Toxicology,* vol. I (New York: Academic Press, 1982), 462. *Aspartame,* ed. L. D. Stegink and L. J. Filer Jr. (New York: Marcel Dekker, 1984), 350, 359. *General and Applied Toxicology,* ed. Bryan Ballantyne, Timothy Marrs, and Paul Turner, vol. 1 (New York: Stockton Press, 1993), 482.

72. Hyman J. Roberts, "Reactions Attributed to Aspartame-Containing Products: 551 cases," *Natural Food & Farming* (March 1992), 23–8.

73. Leon Chaitow, *Thorson's Guide to Amino Acids* (London: Thorson, 1991), 95.

74. Susan C. Smolinske, *Handbook of Food, Drug, and Cosmetic Excipients* (Boca Raton, Fla.: CRC Press, 1992), 236.

75. Bernard Rimland, Ph.D., "The Feingold Diet: An Assessment of the Reviews by Marttes, by Kavale and Forness and Others," *Journal of Learning Disabilities* 16:6 (June/July 1983), 331. (Available from the Autism Research Institute, Publication #51.)

76. Catherine Carrigan, *Healing Depression: A Holistic Guide* (New York: Marlowe and Company, 2000), 1.

77. *Dietary W3 and W6 Fatty Acids: Biological Effects and Nutritional Essentiality,* ed. Claudio Galli and Artemis P. Simopoulos (New York: Kluwer/Plenum, 1989). Claudio Galli and Artemis P. Simopoulos, *Effects of Fatty Acids and Lipids in Health and Disease* (New York: S. Karger, 1994). Joseph Mercola, "Where's the Real Beef?" available on the Internet at www.mercola.com/beef/main.htm.

78. Presenter statement by Andrew Stoll, M.D., in the DAN! (Defeat Autism Now!) 2000 Conference booklet: 8; published by the

Autism Research Institute in San Diego (fax: 619-563-6840 or website: www.autism.com/ari).

79. M. A. Crawford, A. G. Hassam, and P. A. Stevens, "Essential Fatty Acid Requirements in Pregnancy and Lactation with Special Reference to Brain Development," *Prog Lipid Res* 20 (1981), 31–40.

80. "Healing Mood Disorders with Essential Fatty Acids," *Doctors' Prescription for Healthy Living* 4:6, 1.

81. Rhian Edwards, et al., "Omega-3 Polyunsaturated Fatty Acid Levels in the Diet and in Red Blood Cell Membranes of Depressed Patients," *Journal of Affective Disorders* 48 (1998), 149–55. Peter B. Adams, et al., "Arachidonic Acid to Eicosapentaenoic Acid Ratio in Blood Correlates Positively with Symptoms of Depression," *Lipids* 31: suppl (1996), S157–61.

82. Barbara S. Levine. "Most Frequently Asked Questions about DHA," *Nutrition Today* 32 (November/December 1997), 248–9.

83. Kristen A. Bruinsma and Douglas L. Taren, "Dieting, Essential Fatty Acid Intake, and Depression," *Nutrition Reviews* 58 (April 2000), 98–108.

84. Joseph R. Hibbeln, "Fish Consumption and Major Depression," *The Lancet* 351 (April 18, 1998), 1213.

85. Prevention's *New Encyclopedia of Common Diseases* (Emmaus, Pa.: Rodale Press, 1985), 230.

86. H. Beckman, "Phenylalanine in Affective Disorders," *Adv Biol Psychiatry* 10 (1983), 137–47. C. Gibson and A. Gelenberg, "Tyrosine for Depression," *Adv Biol Psychiatry* 10 (1983), 148–59.

87. Michael T. Murray, N.D., *Natural Alternatives to Prozac* (New York: Quill/William Morrow, 1996), 175.

88. Ibid., 118.

89. William Walsh, Ph.D., "The Critical Role of Nutrients in Severe Mental Symptoms," available on the Internet at: www.alternativementalhealth.com/articles/article-pffeiffer.htm.

90. Ronald Hoffman, "Beyond Prozac: Natural Therapies for Anxiety and Depression," *Innovation: The Health Letter of FAIM* (January 31, 1999), 10–11, 13, 15, 17, 19.

91. Catherine Carrigan, *Healing Depression: A Holistic Guide* (New York: Marlowe and Company, 2000), 189.

92. Linda Rector Page, N.D., Ph.D., *Healthy Healing*, (Carmel Valley, Calif.: Healthy Healing Publications, 1997) 103.

93. E. H. Cook and B. L. Leventhal, "The Serotonin System in Autism," *Curr Opin Pediatr* 8:4 (August 1996), 348–54.

94. Syd Baumel, *Dealing with Depression Naturally* (Los Angeles: Keats Publishing, 2000), 12.

95. Ronald Hoffman, "Beyond Prozac: Natural Therapies for Anxiety and Depression," *Innovation: The Health Letter of FAIM* (January 31, 1999), 10–11, 13, 15, 17, 19.

96. Burton Goldberg and the Editors of *Alternative Medicine, Women's Health Series: 2* (Tiburon: Future Medicine Publishing, 1998), 208–209.

97. John R. Lee, M.D., *What Your Doctor May Not Tell You About Menopause* (New York: Warner Books, 1996), 103, 229.

98. Sherry A. Rogers, M.D., *Depression—Cured at Last!* (Sarasota, Fla.: SK Publishing, 1997), 403.

99. Ibid., 408–10.

100. Michael T. Murray, N.D., *Natural Alternatives to Prozac* (New York: Quill/William Morrow, 1996), 56. Sherry A. Rogers, M.D., *Depression—Cured at Last!* (Sarasota, Fla.: SK Publishing, 1997), 144–5.

101. Amy Norton, "Exercise Beats Drugs for Some with Depression," Reuters Health Information (March 28, 2001); available on the Internet at: http://www.nlm.nih.gov/medlineplus/news/fullstory_949.html.

102. P. A. Roos, "Light and Electromagnetic Waves: The Health Implications," *Journal of the Bio-Electro-Magnetics Institute* 3:2 (Summer 1991), 7–12. John Nash Ott, *Health and Light* (Old Greenwich, Conn.: Devin-Adair, 1973).

103. "Learned Optimism More Useful than Truth," available on the Internet at: http://www.globalideasbank.org/1993/1993–38.HTML. R. Liparulo, "Optimists Can Juice Up Your Company's Profit," *Real Estate Today* 28:12 (1995), 5.

## 3: A Model for Healing

104. Richard Leviton, "Migraines, Seizures, and Mercury Toxicity," *Alternative Medicine Digest* 21 (December 1997/January 1998), 61.

## 4: Biological Medicine

105. Unless otherwise indicated, the sources of Dr. Rau's quotes in this chapter are personal communication with the author and a presentation on depression by Dr. Rau at the Education Seminar for European Biological Medicine, sponsored by the Biological Medicine Network at the Marion Foundation in Marion, Mass., May 11–13, 2001.

106. Richard Leviton, "The Ideal Clinic: Arthritis, Parkinson's, and Fibromyalgia," *Alternative Medicine Digest* 13 (June/July 1998), 26.

## 6: Homeopathy

107. Personal communication, 2001. Unless footnoted, quotes throughout this section are from personal communication with Dr. Reichenberg-Ullman.

108. Judyth Reichenberg-Ullman, N.D., L.C.S.W., and Robert Ullman, N.D., *Prozac Free: Homeopathic Alternatives to Conventional Drug Therapies* (Berkeley, Calif.: North Atlantic Books, 2002), xiv.

109. Ibid., xiv.

110. Ibid., 8–12.

111. Ibid., 3–4.

112. Judyth Reichenberg-Ullman, N.D., L.C.S.W., and Robert Ullman, N.D., *Ritalin-Free Kids: Safe and Effective Homeopathic Medicine for ADHD, and Other Behavioral and Learning Problems*, (Roseville, Calif.: Prima Health, 2000), 83.

113. Miranda Castro, R.S.Hom., *The Complete Homeopathy Handbook*, New York: St. Martin's Press, 1990: 3–5. Anne Woodham and David Peters, M.D., *Encyclopedia of Healing Therapies* (New York: Dorling Kindersley, 1997), 126.

114. Judyth Reichenberg-Ullman, N.D., L.C.S.W., and Robert Ullman, N.D., *Ritalin-Free Kids: Safe and Effective Homeopathic Medicine for ADHD, and Other Behavioral and Learning Problems* (Roseville, Calif.: Prima Health, 2000), 95.

115. Ibid., 95–96.

116. Personal communication and Judyth Reichenberg-Ullman, N.D., L.C.S.W., and Robert Ullman, N.D., *Ritalin-Free Kids: Safe*

*and Effective Homeopathic Medicine for ADHD, and Other Behavioral and Learning Problems,* (Roseville, Calif.: Prima Health, 2000), 90.

117. Personal communication and Judyth Reichenberg-Ullman, N.D., L.C.S.W., and Robert Ullman, N.D., *Prozac Free: Homeopathic Alternatives to Conventional Drug Therapies* (Roseville, Calif.: Prima Health, 1999), 57.

## 7: Flower Essence Therapy

118. Patricia Kaminski and Richard Katz, *Flower Essence Repertory* (Nevada City, Calif.: Flower Essence Society, 1996), 3.

119. Edward Bach and F.J. Wheeler, *The Bach Flower Remedies* (New Canaan, Conn.: Keats Publishing, 1977).

120. Patricia Kaminski and Richard Katz, *Flower Essence Repertory* (Nevada City, Calif.: Flower Essence Society, 1996), 5. Patricia Kaminski and Richard Katz, "Using Flower Essences: A Practical Overview" (Nevada City, Calif.,: Flower Essence Society, 1994).

## 8: Soma Therapies

121. Richard Leviton, "Reversing Autism and Depression with Bodywork," *Alternative Medicine* 24 (June/July 1998), 36–41.

122. "CranioSacral Therapy," available at the Upledger Institute Website (http://www.upledger.com/therapies/cst.htm)

123. "What is Osteopathy?" available at the Cranial Academy Website (http://www.cranialacademy.org/whatis.html)

124. "CranioSacral Therapy," available at the Upledger Institute Website (http://www.upledger.com/therapies/cst.htm)

125. Sources: Informational materials of Soma Therapy Centre. Richard Leviton, "Reversing Autism and Depression with Bodywork," *Alternative Medicine* 24 (June/July 1998), 36–41

## 9: Matrix Work and Psychosomatic Medicine

126. Nahoma Asha Clinton, L.C.S.W., Ph.D., "Seemorg Matrix Work, The Transpersonal Energy Psychotherapy," available on the Internet at http://www.matrixwork.org/tara.html.

127. Ibid.

128. Nahoma Asha Clinton, L.C.S.W., Ph.D., "The Story of

SEEMORG," available on the Internet at
http://www.seemorgmatrix.org/seemorg-story.html.

129. Nahoma Asha Clinton, L.C.S.W., Ph.D., "Redefining Trauma," available on the Internet at
http://www.matrixwork.org/manual.htm

## 10: Shamanic and Psychic Healing

130. Richard Leviton, *The Healthy Living Space* (Charlottesville, Va.: Hampton Roads, 2001), 354–8.

131. Ibid., 362–3.

132. Ibid., 364.

133. John Lash, *The Seeker's Handbook* (New York: Harmony Books, 1990), 371.

134. Malidoma Patrice Somé, *Ritual: Power, Healing, and Community* (New York: Penguin, 1997), 12, 19.

135. Malidoma Patrice Somé, *Of Water and the Spirit: Ritual, Magic, And initiation in the Life of an African Shaman* (New York: Penguin, 1994), 9, 10.

# Index

# About the Author

Stephanie Marohn has been writing since she was a child. Her adult writing background is extensive in both journalism and nonfiction trade books. In addition to *Natural Medicine First Aid Remedies* and the six books in the Healthy Mind series (*Natural Medicine Guide to Autism*, with *The Natural Medicine Guide to Depression, The Natural Medicine Guide to Bipolar Disorder, The Natural Medicine Guide to Addiction, The Natural Medicine Guide to Anxiety,* and *The Natural Medicine Guide to Schizophrenia*) she has published more than 30 articles in magazines and newspapers, written two novels and a feature film screenplay, and has had her work included in poetry, prayer, and travel writing anthologies.

Stephanie came to her interest in natural medicine in the way that many people do: through her own healing. For over 10 years, she has relied on natural medicine practitioners for her medical care. Her primary care physician is an acupuncturist and doctor of traditional Chinese medicine. She has also found herbal medicine and homeopathy particularly helpful, and uses both to treat the various maladies of her many animal companions.

Originally from Philadelphia, she has been a resident of the San Francisco Bay Area for over 20 years, and currently lives in Sonoma County, north of the city.

# Hampton Roads Publishing Company

*. . . for the evolving human spirit*

Hampton Roads Publishing Company
publishes books on a variety of subjects,
including metaphysics, health, visionary fiction,
and other related topics.

For a copy of our latest catalog, call toll-free
800-766-8009, or send your name and address to:

Hampton Roads Publishing Company, Inc.
1125 Stoney Ridge Road
Charlottesville, VA 22902

e-mail: hrpc@hrpub.com
www.hrpub.com